KT-492-611

STEP-BY-STEP
DANCE CLASS

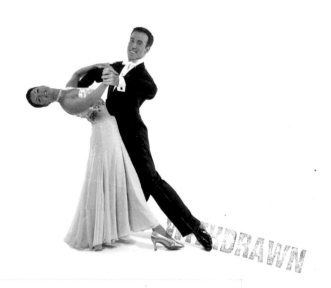

WITHDRAWN

C153838756

KENT LIBRARIES
AND ARCHIVES

C 153838756	
Askews	

10 9 8 7 6 5 4 3 2 1

Published in 2009 by BBC Books, an imprint of Ebury Publishing.
A Random House Group Company

Dance-step instructions © Kele Baker and Ralf Schiller 2009
All other text © Woodlands Books Limited 2009
All series photography © BBC 2009
All other photography © Woodlands Books Limited 2009
Illustrations © Mike Garland

Kele Baker and Ralf Schiller have asserted their right to be identified as the authors of this Work in
accordance with the Copyright, Designs and Patents Act 1988

All rights reserved. No part of this publication may be reproduced, stored in a retrieval system, or
transmitted in any form or by any means, electronic, mechanical, photocopying, recording or otherwise,
without the prior permission of the copyright owner.

The Random House Group Limited Reg. No. 954009

Addresses for companies within the Random House Group can be found at
www.randomhouse.co.uk

A CIP catalogue record for this book is available from the British Library.

ISBN 978 1 846 07765 4

The Random House Group Limited supports the Forest Stewardship Council (FSC), the leading
international forest certification organisation. All our titles that are printed on Greenpeace approved
FSC certified paper carry the FSC logo. Our paper procurement policy can be found at
www.rbooks.co.uk/environment

Commissioning editor: Lorna Russell
Project editor: Laura Higginson
Design: Bobby Birchall, Ana Zeferino-Birchall, Bobby&co
Production controller: Bridget Fish

Colour origination by Altaimage, London
Printed and bound in Germany by Firmengruppe APPL, aprinta druck, Wemding
To buy books by your favourite authors and register for offers, visit www.rbooks.co.uk

The information in this book has been compiled by way of general guidance in relation to dance,
the specific subject addressed, but is not a substitute and not to be relied on for medical, healthcare,
pharmaceutical or other specific professional advice on specific circumstances and in specific locations.
Please make sure you have sufficient space for dancing. Please consult your GP before changing, stopping
or starting any medical treatment and before engaging in any strenuous exercise. So far as the author is
aware the information given is correct and up to date as at December 2009. Practice, laws and regulations
all change, and the reader should obtain up-to-date professional advice on any such issues. The authors
and publishers disclaim, as far as the law allows, any liability arising directly or indirectly from the use, or
misuse, of the information contained in this book.

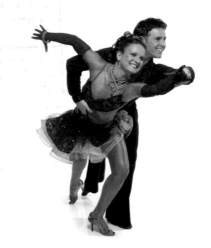

STEP-BY-STEP
DANCE CLASS

DANCE YOURSELF FIT WITH THE BEGINNER'S GUIDE
TO ALL THE DANCES FROM THE SHOW

KELE BAKER AND RALF SCHILLER

BBC
BOOKS

Contents

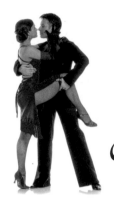

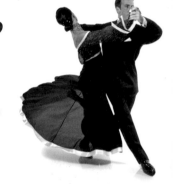

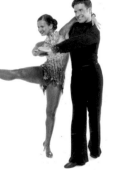

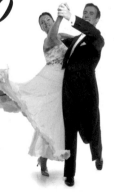

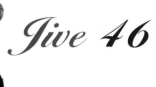

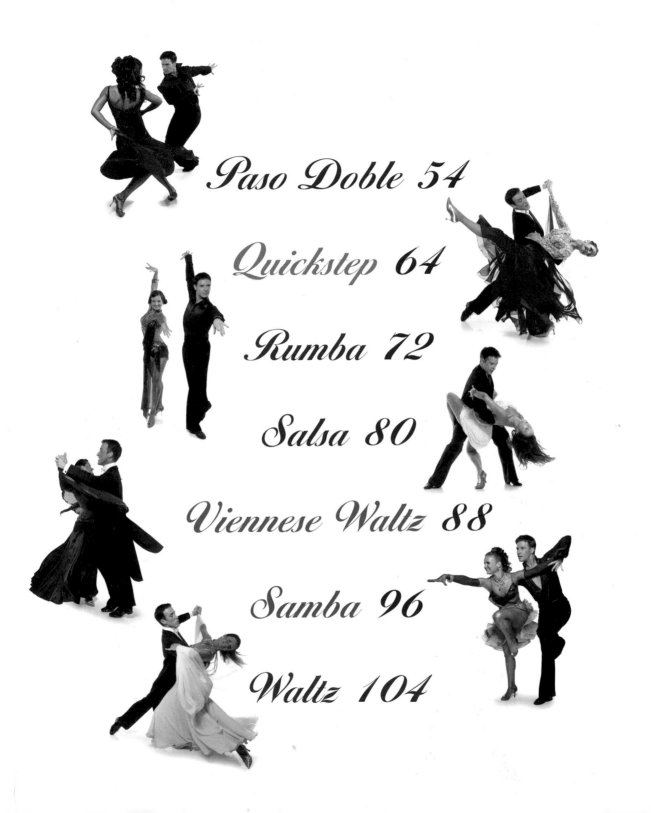

Introduction

For the past five years, millions of viewers have spent their Saturday evenings admiring the glittery rhinestones, elegant tail suits and miles of floating chiffon worn by the brave celebrities who dare to take on the *Strictly Come Dancing* challenge – learning to dance in front of the nation. Along with the glamorous costumes and fantastic live music, viewers revel in tracking the improvement of the celebrity dancers, and the week-by-week development of their skill and confidence.

The 'journey' of these intrepid celebrities (Claudia Winkleman's favourite word on *It Takes Two*) has inspired tens of thousands of others to get up from their couches, venture into dance studios across the country, and embark upon their own dance journey.

DANCE YOURSELF FIT

Dancing is an excellent form of exercise and if done regularly it will lead to improved balance, posture, stamina, core strength and muscle tone – just look at John Sergeant who lost two stone in three months of training for Series Six! Posture and balance improve through controlling the body's movement from one foot to the other, 'pulling up' through the torso, lifting the head, and strengthening the stomach, thighs and bum. Developing this core strength can also help minimize back problems.

Well-defined muscles are a fitness benefit of dancing. Rumba, Cha Cha Cha and Salsa exercise the hips and trim the waist, while 'rise and fall' in the ballroom dances work the calf muscles. Maintaining a wide, toned hold gives your arms and shoulders a workout. Aerobic dances such as Quickstep, Jive, Salsa or Samba improve cardiovascular fitness whilst the slower dances such as the Rumba, Argentine Tango and Waltz require good muscle control, toning the body.

While this book may not offer the high-impact workout of an intensive dance class or an evening of social dancing, it is perfect for those who want to take their first step into dance but haven't yet dared. It provides a safe start, a chance to try the dances in the privacy of your own home, alone or with friends and family.

Hopefully, once your confidence has grown, the big leap from living room to local dance studio will seem less of a grand jeté and more of a gliding chassé. For everyone, this book is full of information on *Strictly*'s 12 competitive dances, wonderful action photos from six series, and *Strictly* professionals Darren Bennett, Lilia Kopylova, Anton du Beke and Erin Boag showing how beginner and advanced figures should look.

THE DIFFERENCE BETWEEN BALLROOM AND LATIN

During all the ballroom dances, which include the Ballroom Tango, Foxtrot, Quickstep, Viennese Waltz and Waltz, the dancers maintain full body contact with the front right half of their bodies (see photo on page 106). Traditionally known as the 'English' style of ballroom dancing, and now known in competitive circles as 'international' or 'standard' style dancing, this is the style danced on *Strictly*. The 'American' style of ballroom dancing is 'American Smooth', in which the couple dance in a side-by-side position as well as in a variety of full-body-contact holds. American Smooth is the thirteenth dance on *Strictly*, but as it utilizes basic steps from the English-style ballroom dances (Ballroom Tango, Foxtrot, Viennese Waltz and Waltz), it hasn't been included in this book.

Latin American dances are performed in a variety of holds as well as in side-by-side position. 'International' style Latin American dances are performed on *Strictly*: Cha Cha Cha, Jive, Rumba, Samba and Paso Doble. There are five 'American' style 'Rhythm' dances: Rumba, Bolero, Cha Cha Cha, Mambo and Swing. American style Rumba is danced to faster music than *Strictly*'s international-style Rumba; the American Cha Cha Cha is danced slower, and both dances have different leg and hip techniques. Swing is similar to Jive, but danced with a different technique and again to slower music. Of the American Rhythm dances, only Mambo and Swing have appeared on *Strictly*, both as exhibition dances.

Salsa is a Latin American dance with its roots in Mambo and Rumba, but it is not included in either international Latin or American Rhythm competitions. Salsa has developed a separate dance community with its own competitions. Argentine Tango is, like Salsa, in a dance world of its own. Argentine Tango has two holds – the 'close embrace' and the 'open hold'. The lead is almost invisibly transmitted and received through the upper body, creating complex patterns of intertwining legs. Argentine Tango is primarily danced socially in Tango clubs ('milongas'), but occasionally it can be seen in stage performances and in specialized Tango competitions.

DRESSING UP FOR THE DANCE FLOOR
Ballroom

In keeping with the free-flowing yet sophisticated nature of ballroom, hair and make-up is glamorous but subtle. Hair may be worn tied up or loose, but not messy. Make-up is usually elegant but natural, with the exception of Ballroom Tango make-up, which may be more dramatic to complement the intensity of the dance.

Latin

For the Latin dances, dark hair and spray tans are the order of the day. Smoky eye make-up looks wonderful for Cha Cha Cha, Rumba, Paso Doble and Salsa, while colourful make-up is more appropriate for Samba and Jive. Argentine Tango style is sultry yet sophisticated – a combination of the ballroom and Latin look. Hair may be worn chic and simple: short and pinned up or loose and wild (although it should not hit the man in the face when turning!). Sparkly accessories add to the glamour.

Taking Your First Steps

Each dance featured in this book comes with step-by-step guides, including illustrations and instructions. The step illustrations are easy-to-follow numbered footprints showing both the man and woman where to place their feet. The instructions describe how to dance each step, and are numbered to correspond with the footprints.

STEP GUIDE TERMS

Ballroom dancing, like most specialized activities, has its own terminology. How often has Len Goodman been heard to say, 'You didn't release your toes on your back steps,' or 'Where were your heel leads?' These terms, as well as others used throughout the book, are explained below.

Closed Hold – Ballroom

The couple face each other, the woman slightly to the man's right, with their bodies lightly touching. The man extends his left arm to the side (the woman her right arm). They clasp hands, but the fingers should not interlock. The clasped hands should be at the eye level of the shorter partner. The man puts his right hand on the woman's left shoulder blade and the woman places her left arm on the man's right arm. The hold should be 'expansive' – arms stretched out with no sagging elbows. Both dancers should keep their shoulders down. The man looks forward and the woman looks left, over the man's right shoulder (see illustration on page 68).

When stepping forward, the right foot steps between the partner's feet. This is called 'in line' and, as it is the normal way of moving, it is not specifically mentioned in the step instructions. Exceptional steps such as 'outside partner' (see opposite page) are mentioned.

Closed Hold – Latin

In Latin closed hold, the man and woman face each other, but their bodies do not touch. The man extends his left arm to the side (the woman her right arm) and they clasp hands (again, no interlocking fingers). The man places his right hand on the woman's shoulder blade, and the woman places her left arm on the man's right arm so that the arms are in full contact. Because the bodies do not touch, there is a more rounded shape to the arms than in the ballroom closed hold (see photo on page 74).

Closed Holds – Argentine Tango

There are two holds for Argentine Tango: 'open hold' and 'close embrace'. The 'open hold' is similar to the Latin closed hold, except that the arms are held lower, about the height of the bottom rib. In the 'close embrace' the man and woman have their weight towards the balls of their feet, so that just their upper bodies touch (but heels are still on the floor). The arms are in a 'low' Latin closed hold, also at the height of the bottom rib, but the man's right arm wraps further around the woman's back. The woman rests her left hand lightly on the man's shoulder or on the back of his neck. The choice of hold depends on the figure and is noted at the beginning of the step instructions (see illustration for holds on page 19).

Single-Hand Hold

The dancers face each other, the man's left hand holding the woman's right hand at about waist level. The upper arms are relaxed and elbows point downwards (see illustration on page 53).

Two-Hand Hold

The two-hand hold is very similar to the single-hand hold, with the addition of the man's right hand holding the woman's left hand.

Promenade Position

The couple's bodies are in a V-shaped position, with the right half of the woman's body tilted slightly away from her partner. The man looks over his left hand and the woman looks over her right hand (see photo on page 106).

Counter-Promenade Position

The couple's bodies are in a V-shaped position, the left half of the woman's body turned slightly away from the man and the right half of the man's body turned slightly away from the woman (the reverse of Promenade Position). The hold is loosened so that the man holds the woman just above her left elbow, and the woman hold the man just above his right elbow (see illustration on page 103).

Outside Partner

Rather than stepping forward with the right foot between the partner's feet (see Closed Hold – Ballroom on opposite page), the dancer's right leg moves forward just outside the partner's right hip (see illustration on page 42). In this book, outside partner is most frequently danced on the partner's right side, so the side is not indicated in the instructions. In Argentine Tango, outside partner is danced on both the right and left sides, so the side is indicated.

Forward, Backward and Side Steps – Ballroom

When walking or dancing, the leg you are standing on is the 'supporting leg', and the leg in transition from one step to the next is the 'moving leg'.

A forward step, particularly the first step of a figure, is taken with a 'heel lead'. As with normal walking, first the heel touches the ground, then the whole foot, then the heel lifts up as the body weight moves forward into the next step.

In backward walks the leg swings out first, keeping the toe of the moving leg in contact with the floor. As the body moves backward, the weight is transferred first to the toe then on to the whole foot, including the heel. The toe of the supporting leg lifts off the floor as the moving leg moves behind the supporting leg.

For side steps, the moving leg steps either to the left or right, away from the supporting leg.

Forward, Backward and Side Steps – Latin

In all steps, the big toe of the moving foot remains in contact with the floor as each step is taken on the ball of the foot first, followed by the whole foot ('ball flat'). The exception is Paso Doble, in which the leg and foot action is the same as in the ballroom dances, with 'heel leads' on the forward steps and released toes on the backward steps.

The Latin American dances differ in their techniques for the use of the knees. For Rumba and Cha Cha Cha, each step is taken on to a straight leg. In Jive, the dancer's knee starts bent and ends straight on steps 1, 2, 5 and 8. On steps 3 and 6 the knee stays bent, and on steps 4 and 7 the knee is relaxed. In Samba, the dancer steps on to a bent knee on all the numbered beats, and steps on to a straight knee on all the 'a' beats (see Music on page 11).

Forward and Backward Steps – Argentine Tango

The man steps forward with a 'heel lead' or 'ball flat' (a matter of personal style). The woman steps forward 'ball flat'. For the backward steps, both the man and woman keep the toe of the supporting foot in contact with the floor as the weight transfers to the back foot (the opposite to the ballroom dances). On all steps the inside of the moving foot brushes past the inside of the supporting foot.

Heel turn

As weight is transferred to the heel during a backward step, the body turns, pivoting on the heel. While turning, the moving leg is drawn backwards to meet the supporting leg (the legs should meet only when the full amount of turn has been made). When the legs are together, weight is then transferred from the supporting leg to the moving leg – this step is taken 'in place'.

Rise and Fall

The Foxtrot, Quickstep, Viennese Waltz and Waltz have a characteristic 'rise and fall', an up-and-down pattern, in which the knees bend and straighten, with some steps being danced on the toes. Only two ballroom dances do not have 'rise and fall': Ballroom Tango (danced with slightly flexed knees throughout) and Argentine Tango (danced at a normal walking level).

Start with knees comfortably flexed. Straighten the knees without locking them. Slowly rise up on to the toes then lower the heels to the floor. Complete the movement by flexing the knees again. Practice rise and fall first standing on both feet, then on one foot at a time. How high to rise on the toes varies from dance to dance. As it is quite an advanced technique, it is not covered in this book.

The rise and fall is given for each figure at the end of the step instructions, using the following notations:
Heel or Heel-Flat – start with a 'heel lead', then the whole foot touches the floor
Heel-Toe – start with a 'heel lead', then rise on to toes
Toe – on to toes
Toe-Heel – start on toes, then lower heel to floor finally flexing knee
Toe-Flat – start on toes, then lower heel to floor
Ball – partial weight on the ball of foot, no rise – (for Paso Doble only: step with small rise)

Ball-Heel or Ball-Flat – start on the ball of foot, then lower heel

Whole foot – place whole foot on the floor

TRAVELLING AROUND THE FLOOR

The travelling dances (Argentine Tango, Ballroom Tango, Foxtrot, Quickstep, Samba, Paso Doble, Viennese Waltz and Waltz) move anticlockwise around the dance floor. For the figures in these dances, the nearest edge of the dance floor is always the right side of the step illustrations.

Leading and Following

It is the nature of ballroom and Latin American dancing that the man leads and the woman follows. It's not sexist – it's just how the dances evolved. While it is very helpful for the woman to know her steps, it is the responsibility of the man to move his body in a helpful fashion so that the woman feels what she must do next. The woman then moves her body in response to the direction given. If the man gives the 'lead' at the right time, both the man and the woman will be able to dance their steps together and in time to the music.

MUSIC

Each style of music has its own rhythm. The most common rhythmic pattern in western music has four beats – one strong beat followed by three weak beats. This musical rhythm is applicable to most ballroom and Latin dances. Viennese Waltz and Waltz have three beats – one strong beat and two weak beats. Argentine Tango, Ballroom Tango

and Paso Doble have two beats – one strong beat followed by one weak beat. The rhythmic pattern for dance steps is the 'timing'. Timing is interwoven into the musical rhythm and is therefore unique to each dance. Timing will be discussed further throughout the book. The timing for each step is given in brackets in the instructions. The various timings are:

Quick

One beat of music – written as (Q) or in numerical form (1, 2, 3, etc.).

Slow

Two beats of music, with the step taken on the first beat and no step taken on the second beat – written as (S) or in numerical form (e.g. 4 'hold' 1).

&

A step occurring halfway in between two beats. Cha Cha Cha, for example, is full of '&' beats.

a

An 'a' beat is similar to an '&' beat, occurring in between two beats, but the 'a' beat is taken closer to the second beat. In Samba, the 'a' beat is taken ¾ of the way between the first beat and the second beat. In Jive, the 'a' beat is taken ⅔ of the way between the first beat and the second beat.

SUGGESTED AMALGAMATIONS

Included in each step-by-step guide is a list of possible orders in which to dance the figures. When you've mastered the figures, why not invent your own amalgamations?

Argentine Tango

The Argentine Tango's mood is intimate, conveying desire, jealousy and passion. Originating in the bars and clubs of late nineteenth-century Buenos Aires, it is a dance that is subtle in the upper body, with the dramatic action of Ochos and Ganchos going on in the legs and feet. There is no set timing for figures; slows and quicks are led by the man as he interprets the music. Unlike other dances, the woman is occasionally allowed to control the timing, making the Argentine Tango a 'dance dialogue'. With influences from Europe, the Caribbean, South America and Africa, the Tango has developed into one of the most global of dances.

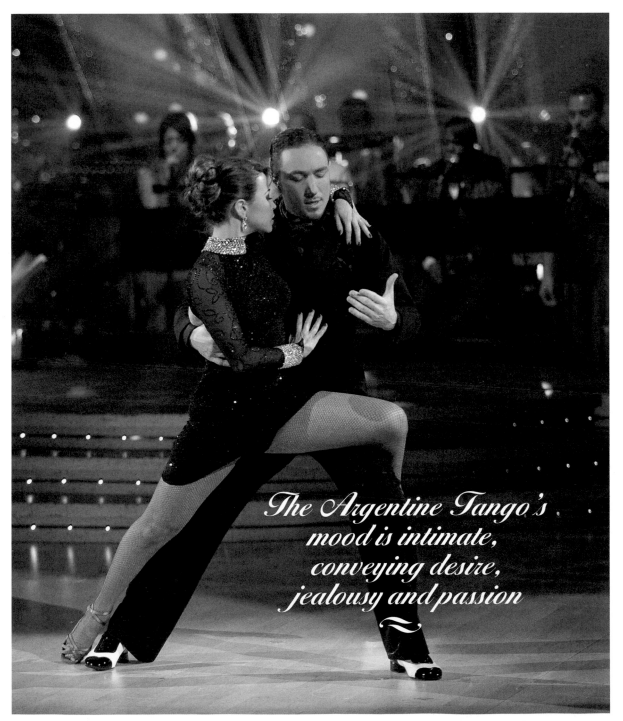

The Argentine Tango's mood is intimate, conveying desire, jealousy and passion
~

The Dance

INCLINADA (TILT)
In this Inclinada, the woman's right leg hooks over the man's left hip while the man lunges to his left. Notice how the hold can change to suit the different shapes and figures.

CALESITA (CAROUSEL)
The woman is lifted on to the toes of one foot, and makes small 'decorations' with her free leg. The man moves around the woman, turning her while she remains balanced.

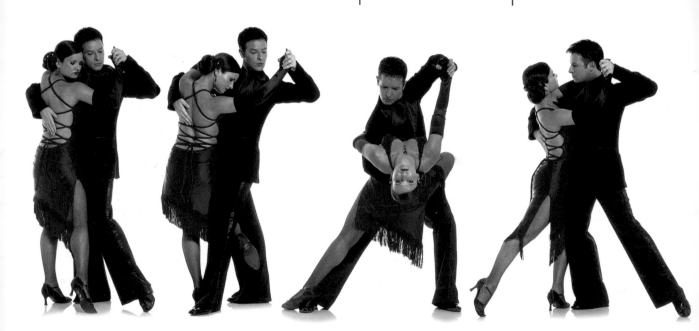

ABRAZO (THE EMBRACE)
The close embrace is cheek to cheek, with the bodies making an upside-down 'V'. The hold can also be wider, with the dancers upright, allowing space for fancier figures.

GANCHO (HOOK)
The Gancho is a flick of the lower leg in between the partner's legs. The thighs and calf muscles connect, making this a flirtatious move requiring coordination.

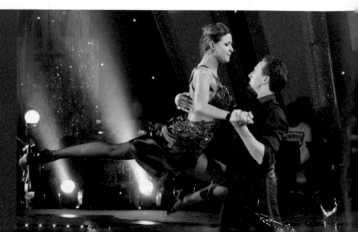

LEN'S OVERVIEW

The dancers should only have eyes for each other, dancing is if there's no-one else in the room. The Argentine Tango is more authentic than Ballroom Tango, closer to what was danced in the brothels of Buenos Aires in the nineteenth century. It's an improvised, sexy dance that moves to the rhythm of the music. It is less aggressive than the Ballroom Tango, right down to the dancers' expressions, which should show passion rather than contempt. The judges are looking for intricate footwork, stunning lines, plenty of musicality and a dramatic, emotional relationship between the dancers.

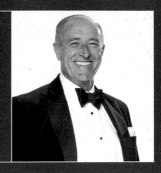

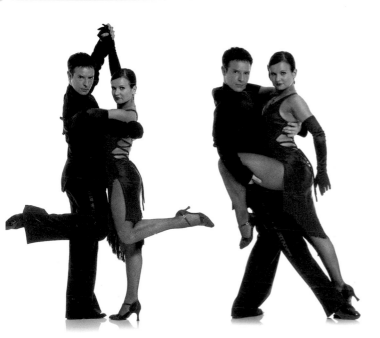

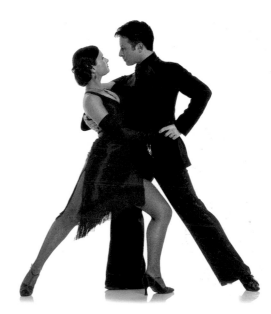

SYMMETRICAL POSE

A classic position from the early days of Argentine Tango. The couple's outstretched arms are lifted high above their heads, and the raised lower legs are reminiscent of the 1920s.

LUNGE WITH LEG UP

An exotic line that is pure Argentine Tango. The woman's leg is over the man's hip as he lunges backward. The man could hold the woman's leg or, alternatively, caress her hair.

PROFILE LINE

The hold is more casual as the man lowers his left arm, bringing the woman's hand to his hip. The couple's thighs are touching, and there is eye-to-eye contact.

EXTREME LUNGE

The intensity of this dance allows the position to go close to the ground. The extended arms can be taken above the head for dramatic presentation.

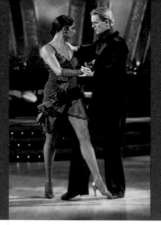

OCHO ADELANTE (FORWARD OCHO)

The man leads the woman into provocative forward swivels. He can remain still or execute intricate footwork while the woman is swivelling. Ochos can also be danced backward (Ochos Atras).

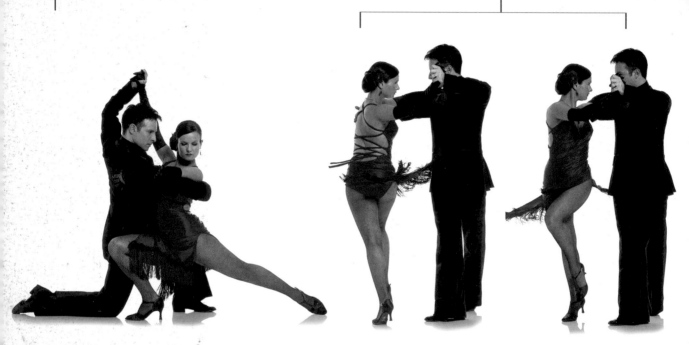

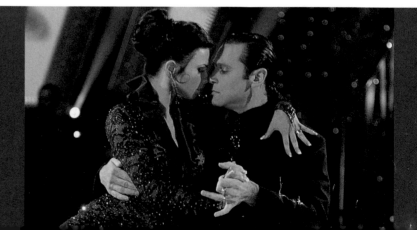

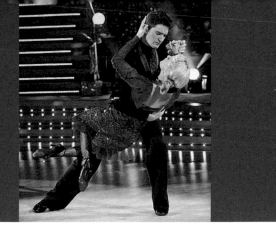

The key to the Argentine Tango is passion, demonstrated through rhythmic walking, intricate intertwining legs and dramatic lines. The hold is flexible, allowing for variety in movement and mood.

TIMING

Argentine Tango music is written either as one heavy and one light beat, or one heavy and three light beats. The couple can choose to dance the steps as 'slows' or 'quicks'. Try dancing all steps as 'slows', then experiment with changing two consecutive steps to 'quicks'. All Ochos should be danced as slows.

MUSIC

The music is in either 2/4 or 4/4 rhythm, but the tone is more subtle than Ballroom Tango. The bandoneón, a small accordion, is the 'voice' of Tango. Traditional songs include 'La Cumparsita' and 'El Choclo', while the most-recognized modern Tango music comes from the group Gotan Project.

HOLD & POSTURE

The hold can vary, from a cheek-to-cheek embrace for rhythmic walking patterns ('La Caminita'), to an open hold with space between the couple for fancier figures such as Ochos Adelante, Ochos Atras and Ganchos.

LEGS & FEET

The sexiness of the dance is expressed mostly through the lower body, so elegant and precise use of legs and feet is desirable – great-looking shoes really help!

DRESS

Dress to impress: a sexy dress or skirt with a slit up the right side for her; a suit with tie or cravat for him.

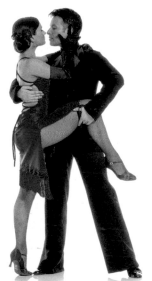 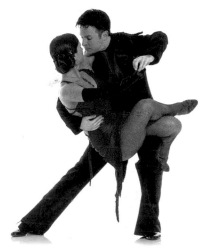

PASSION

Every aspect of this pose demonstrates pure Argentine Tango desire – the close embrace, her confident posture while he holds her leg provocatively, the intense eye contact and the caressing of his face.

SENTADA

An advanced position in which the man shows his strength. The woman is sitting on the man's left knee as if she were sitting in a chair. The pose can be upright or inclined.

The Steps

SALIDA
MAN'S STEPS

This figure can be danced in open hold or close embrace.

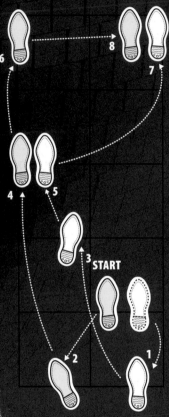

Start with feet together, weight on left foot
1 Right foot back
2 Left foot side
3 Right foot forward outside partner on lady's right side
4 Left foot forward
5 Right foot closes to left foot
6 Left foot forward
7 Right foot side
8 Left foot closes to right foot
End with feet together, weight on left foot

Notes

Steps 6–8 may turn up to ¼ to left.

When starting with the Salida at the beginning of the dance, it is polite to start with step 2, so the man does not accidentally step backward into another dancer.

There is no rise and fall in Argentine Tango. The technique for forward and backward walking is described in the Introduction (see page 10).

SALIDA
LADY'S STEPS

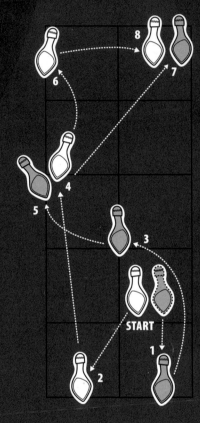

Start with feet together, weight on right foot
1 Left foot forward
2 Right foot side
3 Left foot back
4 Right foot back
5 Left foot crosses in front of right foot ('The Cross')
6 Right foot back
7 Left foot side
8 Right foot closes to left foot
End with feet together, weight on right foot

ROCK STEP AND FORWARD OCHO
MAN'S STEPS

This figure can be danced in open hold or close embrace.

Start with feet together, weight on left foot
1 Right foot back
2 Left foot side
3 Right foot forward outside partner on lady's right side
4 Left foot forward
5 Replace weight back on to right foot
6 Left foot back (small step) just behind right foot – then turn shoulders to the right to lead lady to swivel
7 Right foot closes next to left foot, then turn shoulders to the left to lead lady to swivel, ending in original hold
8–10 Salida steps 6–8
End with feet together, weight on left foot

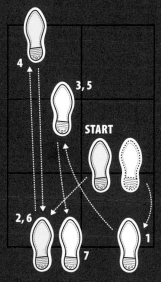

ROCK STEP AND FORWARD OCHO
LADY'S STEPS

Start with feet together, weight on right foot
1 Left foot forward
2 Right foot side
3 Left foot back
4 Right foot back
5 Replace weight forward on to left foot
6 Right foot forward in line with left foot, outside partner on man's right side. When man turns his shoulders, swivel on right foot to the right, ending with left hip closer to man
7 Left foot forward in front of man. When man turns his shoulders, swivel on left foot to the left, ending in original hold
8–10 Salida steps 6–8
End with feet together, weight on right foot

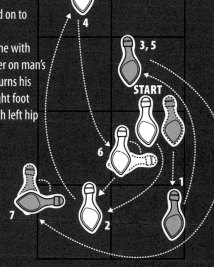

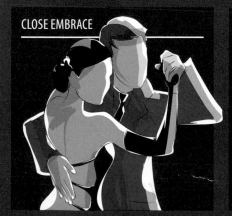

CLOSE EMBRACE

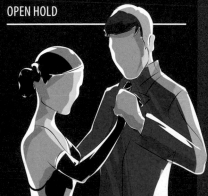

OPEN HOLD

SUGGESTED AMALGAMATIONS

Salida – Rock Step and Forward Ocho
Salida – Back Ocho with Gancho
Salida – Cambio de Frente
Salida – Rock Step and Forward Ocho – Back Ocho with Gancho – Cambio de Frente

The Steps

BACK OCHO WITH GANCHO
MAN'S STEPS

This figure is danced in open hold.

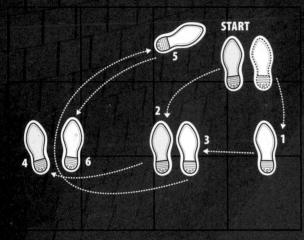

Start with feet together, weight on left foot
1 Right foot back
2 Left foot side
3 Right foot closes to left foot ('Traspie') – then turn shoulders to left to lead lady to swivel
4 Left foot side, then turn shoulders to the right to lead lady to swivel
5 When lady has stepped back, step right foot diagonally forward, right knee slightly bent, between lady's legs and closer to her right foot
6 Replace weight on to left foot and close right foot next to left foot – then turn shoulders to the left to lead lady to swivel, ending in original hold
7–9 Salida steps 6–8
End with feet together, weight on left foot

BACK OCHO WITH GANCHO
LADY'S STEPS

Start with feet together, weight on right foot
1 Left foot forward
2 Right foot side
3 When man turns his shoulders, swivel on right foot to the left, ending with right hip closer to man and left foot next to right foot without weight
4 Left foot back then, when man turns his shoulders, swivel on left foot to the right, ending with left hip closer to man ('Back Ocho')
5 Right foot back then, when man's leg is between lady's legs, flick lower left leg back between man's legs, so that left calf muscle touches momentarily against underside of man's right thigh ('Gancho')
6 Left foot forward in front of man – when man turns his shoulders, swivel on left foot to the left, ending in original hold
7–9 Salida steps 6–8
End with feet together, weight on right foot

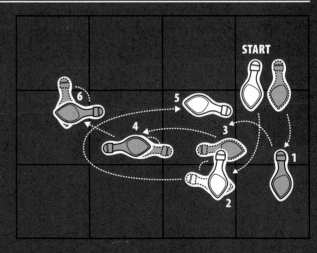

CAMBIO DE FRENTE
MAN'S STEPS

This figure can be danced in open hold or close embrace.

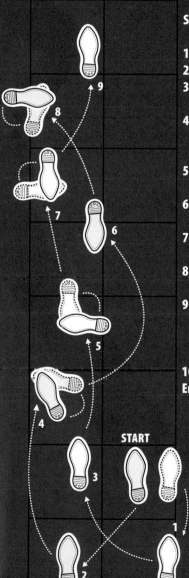

Start with feet together, weight on left foot
1 Right foot back
2 Left foot side
3 Right foot forward outside partner on lady's right side
4 Left foot forward and slightly between lady's feet – start to turn to left
5 Right foot to side, continue to turn left
6 Left foot back, having turned ½ to left over steps 4–6
7 Right foot back and slightly side, continue to turn left
8 Left foot side, continue to turn left
9 Right foot forward outside partner on lady's right side, having turned ½ to left over steps 7–9
10–14 Salida steps 4–8
End with feet together, weight on left foot

CAMBIO DE FRENTE
LADY'S STEPS

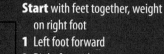

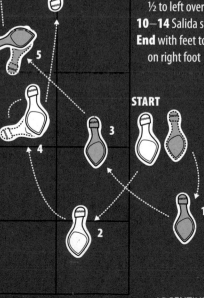

Start with feet together, weight on right foot
1 Left foot forward
2 Right foot side
3 Left foot back
4 Right foot back and slightly side – start to turn to left
5 Left foot side, continue to turn to left
6 Right foot forward outside partner on man's right side, having turned ½ to left over steps 4–6
7 Left foot forward and slightly between man's feet, continue to turn left
8 Right foot side, continue to turn left
9 Left foot back, having turned ½ to left over steps 7–9
10–14 Salida steps 4–8
End with feet together, weight on right foot

Ballroom Tango

In Ballroom Tango, slow, deliberate 'stalking' walks and severe lines alternate with sudden, fast staccato movement, giving the dance its light and shade. Emerging from the ghettos of Argentina in the 1890s, the dance migrated to Europe in the twentieth century, where it was cleaned up and became a pre-War craze – although it never lost its shady reputation. Development of the dance and music in Germany in the 1930s gave what is now the Ballroom Tango its strength and intensity. This is an aggressive yet sexy dance that stirs up real excitement when danced with the control and power it demands.

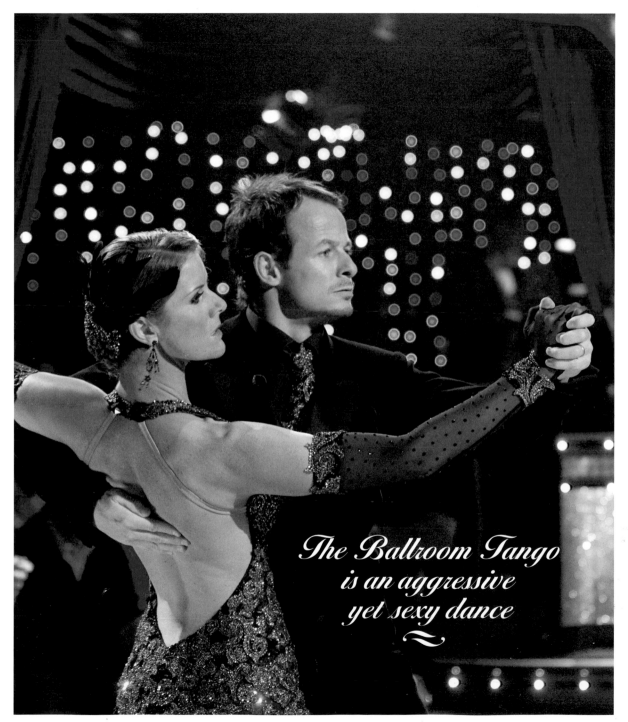

*The Ballroom Tango
is an aggressive
yet sexy dance*

The Dance

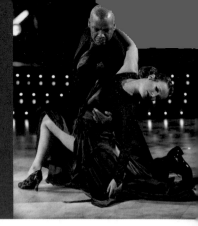

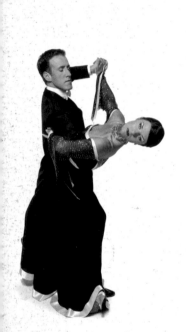

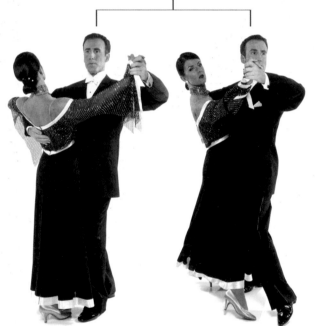

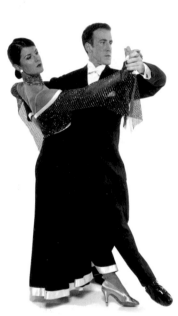

CONTRA CHECK
A perfect expression of the passionate nature of the Ballroom Tango. The man dominates the woman, leading her to lean away from him with her head and shoulders.

TANGO HOLD
This is much more compact than basic ballroom hold. Anton's right arm is further around Erin's body, and her left hand is underneath his armpit (inset).

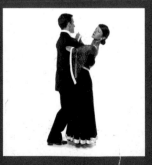

STALKING WALKS
Elongated steps take the dancers across the floor with cat-like grace. The taut attitude of the bodies and the stern facial expressions are key to the character of the dance.

LEN'S OVERVIEW

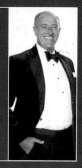

The Ballroom Tango is an aggressive dance. There's not much smiling, but there's a lot of sexy seduction. Don't forget that it has its roots in a dance performed by Argentine gauchos and prostitutes. While the Waltz and Foxtrot are gliding dances, the Ballroom Tango is flat and staccato, with sharp foot and head movements performed at lightning speed. Most dances are soft and flowing, but the Ballroom Tango goes in big blips, like a heart monitor on a screen. It can be ugly if you do it badly, but, done properly, it's tremendously exciting.

Ballroom Tango should be danced with both stalking and staccato walks, and sharp head and body movements. Slightly flexed knees and strong, quick steps mean the Ballroom Tango is a good leg workout.

TIMING

Ballroom Tango music has one heavy and one light beat. 'Slows' are danced on the heavy beat only, and two 'quicks' are danced together on the heavy and light beats. Each figure has its own combination of 'slows' and 'quicks', making this a dance of considerably varied timing.

MUSIC

The music is in 2/4 time, giving it a marching beat, and the speed is 32 bars per minute. 'Maneater' by Nelly Furtado or the traditional song 'Jealousy' evoke the rhythm of this dance.

HOLD & POSTURE

The hold is compact, with arms less outstretched than in the other ballroom dances. The man holds his partner closer to him, allowing him to whisk the woman very quickly into dramatic positions.

LEGS & FEET

The knees are slightly flexed throughout, and there is no rise and fall. The feet are placed on each step – no gliding. Judges are looking for expressive slow and quick steps, and snappy changes of direction.

DRESS

A tail suit may be changed for a more lounge-like shorter jacket, reminiscent of Ballroom Tango's informal roots. Erin wears alluring and dramatic black and silver satin.

SPANISH DRAG

The woman starts in a deep line. The man slowly brings her up, then suddenly they both drop into a promenade position to continue their progress across the floor.

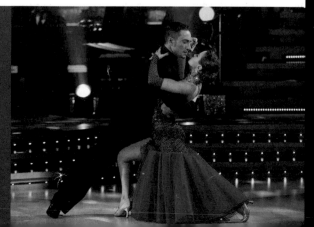

The Steps

TWO WALKS
MAN'S STEPS

This figure is danced in closed hold.

Start with weight on right foot
1 Left foot forward (S)
2 Right foot forward (S)
End with weight on right foot
(1. Heel, 2. Heel)

TWO WALKS
LADY'S STEPS

Start with weight on left foot
1 Right foot back (S)
2 Left foot back (S)
End with weight on left foot
(1. Ball-Heel, 2. Ball-Heel)

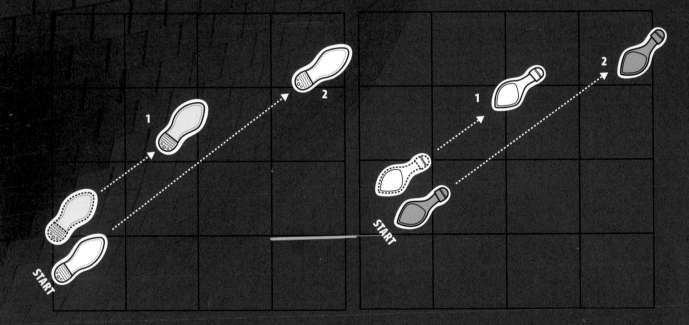

SUGGESTED AMALGAMATIONS

Two Walks – Progressive Side Step
Two Walks – Rock Turn
Two Walks – Link and Closed Promenade
Two Walks – Progressive Side Step – Rock Turn – Two Walks
    – Link and Closed Promenade

PROGRESSIVE SIDE STEP
MAN'S STEPS

This figure is danced in closed hold.

Start with weight on right foot
1 Left foot forward (Q)
2 Right foot side (small step) (Q)
End with weight on right foot
(1. Heel, 2. Whole foot)

PROGRESSIVE SIDE STEP
LADY'S STEPS

Start with weight on left foot
1 Right foot back (Q)
2 Left foot side (small step) (Q)
End with weight on left foot
(1. Ball-Heel, 2. Whole foot)

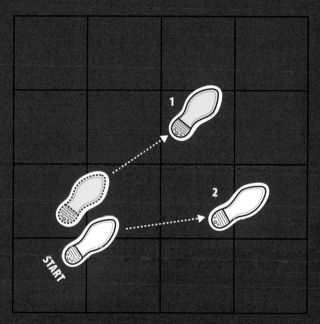

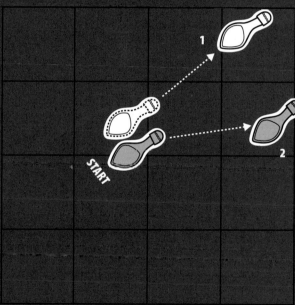

The Steps

ROCK TURN
MAN'S STEPS

This figure is danced in closed hold.

Start with weight on right foot
1 Left foot forward (S)
2 Turn ⅛ to right, then right foot forward (S)
3 Turn ⅛ to right, then left foot back (Q)
4 Replace weight forward on to right foot (Q)
5 Replace weight back on to left foot (S)
6 Right foot back (Q)
7 Turn ¼ to left, then left foot side (small step) (Q)
8 Right foot closes to left foot (S)
End with weight on right foot
(1. Heel, 2. Heel, 3. Ball-Heel, 4. Ball-Heel, 5. Ball-Heel, 6. Ball-Heel,
7. Whole foot; 8. Whole foot)

ROCK TURN
LADY'S STEPS

Start with weight on left foot
1 Right foot back (S)
2 Turn ⅛ to right, then left foot back (S)
3 Turn ⅛ to right, then right foot forward (Q)
4 Replace weight back on to left foot (Q)
5 Replace weight forward on to right foot (S)
6 Left foot forward (Q)
7 Turn ¼ to left, then right foot side (Q)
8 Left foot closes to right foot (S)
End with weight on left foot
(1. Ball-Heel, 2. Ball-Heel, 3. Heel, 4. Ball-Heel, 5. Heel, 6. Heel,
7. Whole foot, 8. Whole foot)

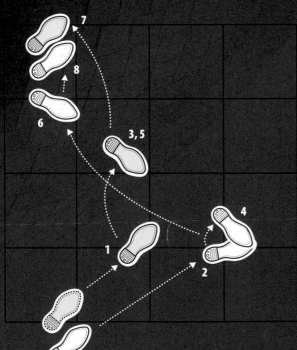

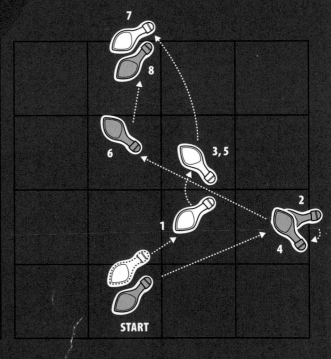

LINK AND CLOSED PROMENADE
MAN'S STEPS

This figure is danced in closed hold.

Start with weight on right foot
1 Left foot forward (Q)
2 Turn shoulders to right to turn lady to promenade position, then right foot side (small step) (Q)
3 Left foot side in promenade position (S)
4 Right foot forward and across in promenade position (Q)
5 Turn shoulders slightly to left to resume original hold, then left foot side (small step) (Q)
6 Right foot closes to left foot (S)
End with weight on right foot
(1. Heel, 2. Ball-Heel, 3. Heel, 4. Heel, 5. Whole foot, 6. Whole foot)

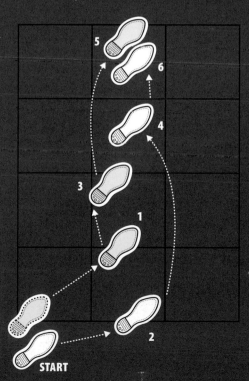

LINK AND CLOSED PROMENADE
LADY'S STEPS

Start with weight on left foot
1 Right foot back (Q)
2 Turn ¼ to right to promenade position, then left foot side (Q)
3 Right foot side in promenade position (S)
4 Left foot forward and across in promenade position (Q)
5 Turn ¼ to left to resume original hold, then right foot side (Q)
6 Left foot closes to right foot (S)
End with weight on left foot
(1. Ball-Heel, 2. Ball-Heel, 3. Heel, 4. Heel, 5. Whole foot, 6. Whole foot)

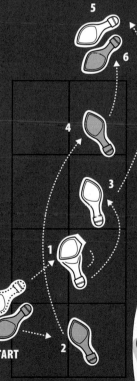

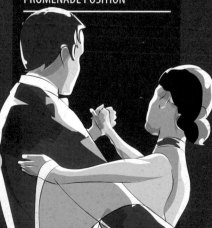

BALLROOM TANGO HOLD IN PROMENADE POSITION

Cha Cha Cha

As the name suggests, the Cha Cha Cha is a little number that allows the dancers a bit of fun and a lot of flirting. The Cha Cha Cha and the Rumba, both from Cuba, share similar step patterns, but the mood could not be more different. While the Rumba is about seduction, the Cha Cha Cha is light-hearted, with the couple playfully enjoying each other's company. During the 1940s, everyone was dancing Mambo, but it was fast and very difficult to dance. Orchestras started to slow down the music, and a new dance with a syncopated rhythm was born.

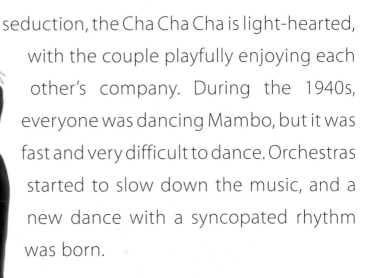

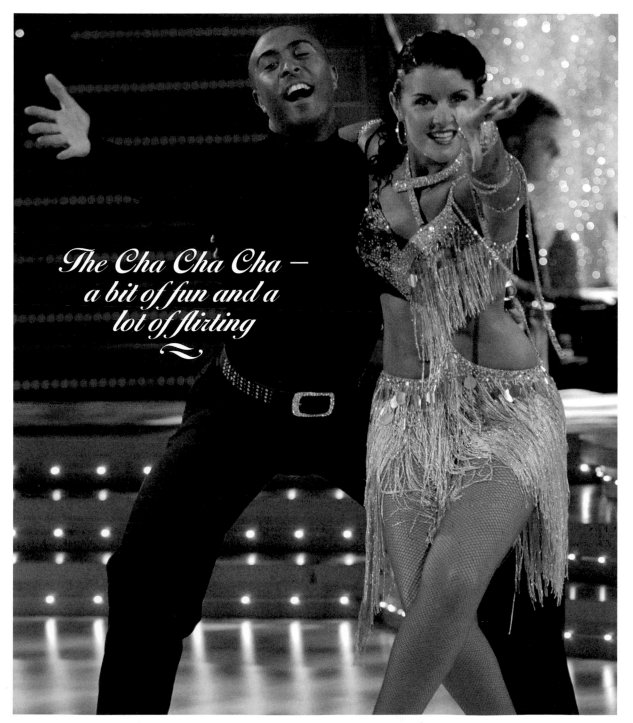

*The Cha Cha Cha –
a bit of fun and a
lot of flirting*

The Dance

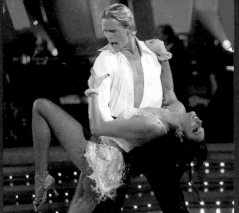

OPEN HIP TWIST
Lilia has danced the first of the Open Hip Twist's two half-turns, made more challenging by dancing it in 'handshake hold'. It's a difficult figure in which to maintain balance.

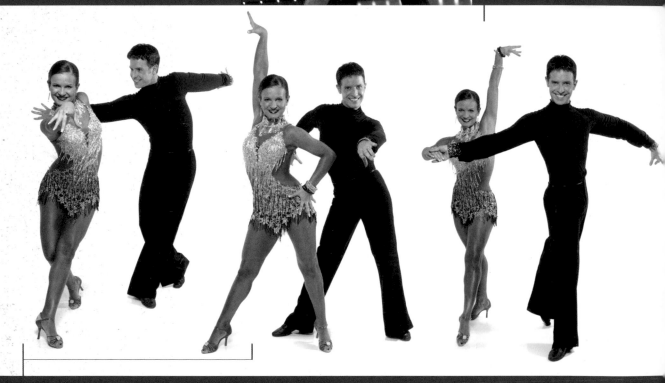

CUBAN BREAK
Cuban Break is a group of rapid steps in which the dancers cross and uncross their legs repeatedly. The arms are free and expressive, and there's an emphasis on the syncopated rhythm.

LEN'S OVERVIEW

The Cha Cha Cha is a gay dance, in the old-fashioned sense of the word. It's sexy, but never in the same 'serious' way as the Tango or the Rumba. It's important for me to see that the couple are enjoying themselves. I'm looking for a sense of spontaneity although, of course, the steps are very difficult and have to be done precisely. It's extremely important that the dancers know where their partner's body weight is going to be.

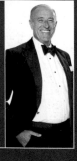

FAN

Fan appears in both Cha Cha Cha and Rumba, but the attitude is cheekier in Cha Cha Cha. After forming this perpendicular position, the woman closes her feet, then steps forward towards the man.

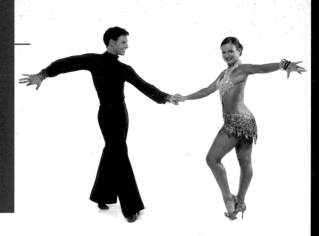

Cha Cha Cha is characterized by a playful interchange between the man and woman. The mood is light and sexy. It's a very cardiovascular dance with lots of quick steps.

TIMING

Like the Rumba and Salsa, the Cha Cha Cha is a dance to four-beat music that has a strong first beat. Cha Cha Cha has a half beat between the fourth beat and the next first beat. Three Cha Cha Cha steps are danced on beats '4&1'. There are two ways to start dancing with the music: either count with the music '1234&1' then start with step one of the figure, or count '123', dance a Cha Cha Cha on '4&1' then dance step one of the figure.

MUSIC

'Sway' is classic Cha Cha Cha, recorded by performers from Rosemary Clooney to Pussycat Dolls. Duffy's 'Mercy' has perfect character, as does 'Kiss', the Tom Jones version. Cha Cha Cha speed is 32 bars per minute.

HOLD & POSTURE

Cha Cha Cha requires a strong, toned upper body, with good connection between the partners and free, playful hips and legs expressing the rhythm of the dance.

LEGS & FEET

Legs are turned out and toes are pressed firmly into the floor, helping to create the teasing Cha Cha Cha hip movement.

DRESS

Dresses are generally short and revealing, and have caused Bruce to ask, 'What aren't you wearing?' on more than one occasion. Sparkle and fringing enhance the effect of sharp movements, hip action and changes of direction. Men wear an open-front shirt showing a bit of chest, or a tight top to show body shape.

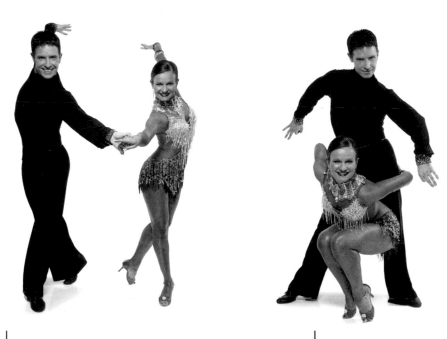

NEW YORK

Pioneer Cha Cha Cha dancers Pierre and Lavelle discovered this move in the clubs of New York. The feet are turned out, and there's a strong 'V' shape through the bodies and outstretched arms.

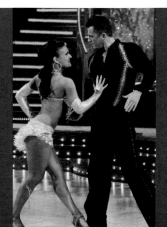

WIGGLE

A typically sassy Cha Cha Cha movement. The man's position is strong and macho. The woman crouches at his feet, holding on to his hips, then wiggles her way up his legs.

The Steps

BASIC STEP
MAN'S STEPS

This figure is danced in closed hold or two-hand hold.

Start with weight on right foot
1 Left foot forward (2)
2 Replace weight back on to right foot (3)
3 Left foot side (small step) (4)
4 Right foot closes to left foot (&)
5 Left foot side (1)
6 Right foot back (2)
7 Replace weight forward on to left foot (3)
8 Right foot side (small step) (4)
9 Left foot closes to right foot (&)
10 Right foot side (1)
End with weight on right foot
(Ball-Flat on all steps)

BASIC STEP
LADY'S STEPS

Start with weight on left foot
1 Right foot back (2)
2 Replace weight forward on to left foot (3)
3 Right foot side (small step) (4)
4 Left foot closes to right foot (&)
5 Right foot side (1)
6 Left foot forward (2)
7 Replace weight back on to right foot (3)
8 Left foot side (small step) (4)
9 Right foot closes to left foot (&)
10 Left foot side (1)
End with weight on left foot
(Ball-Flat on all steps)

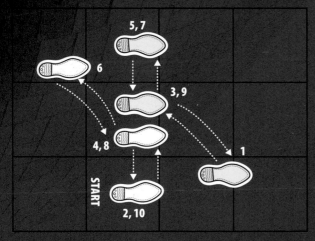

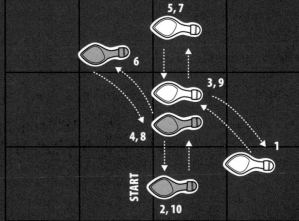

Note

This figure turns gently to left, and may turn up to ½.

Always start with a Basic Step, then proceed to another figure.

NEW YORKS
MAN'S STEPS

This figure is danced from closed hold or two-hand hold.

Start with feet apart, weight on right foot

1 Release hold with right hand, turn ¼ to right, then left foot forward (2)
2 Replace weight back on to right foot (3)
3 Turn ¼ to left to face lady, take two-hand hold, then left foot side (small step) (4)
4 Right foot closes to left foot (&)
5 Left foot side (1)
6 Release hold with left hand, turn ¼ to left, then right foot forward (2)
7 Replace weight back on to left foot (3)
8 Turn ¼ to right to face lady, take two-hand hold, then right foot side (small step) (4)
9 Left foot closes to right foot (&)
10 Right foot side (1)
End with weight on right foot
(Ball-Flat on all steps)

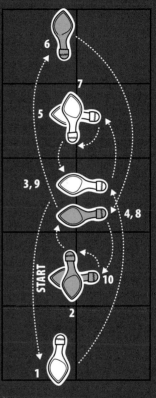

SUGGESTED AMALGAMATIONS

Basic Step – Spot Turns
Basic Step – Time Step
Basic Step – New Yorks – repeat New Yorks steps 1–5 –
   Spot Turns steps 6–10
Basic Step – New Yorks – repeat New Yorks steps 1–5 –
   Spot Turns steps 6–10 – Time Step

NEW YORKS
LADY'S STEPS

Start with feet apart, weight on left foot

1 Turn ¼ to left, then right foot forward (2)
2 Replace weight back on to left foot (3)
3 Turn ¼ to right to face man, then right foot side (small step) (4)
4 Left foot closes to right foot (&)
5 Right foot side (1)
6 Turn ¼ to right, then left foot forward (2)
7 Replace weight back on to right foot (3)
8 Turn ¼ to left to face man, then left foot side (small step) (4)
9 Right foot closes to left foot (&)
10 Left foot side (1)
End with weight on left foot
(Ball-Flat on all steps)

Note

If starting New York in closed hold, then man's right arm releases lady on preceding 'Cha Cha Cha'.

See illustration of New York step 1 on page 33

There are two ways to start dancing with the music: either count with the music '1234&1' then start with step one of the figure, or count '123', dance a Cha Cha Cha on '4&1' then dance step one of the figure.

The Steps

SPOT TURNS
MAN'S STEPS

This figure is danced from closed hold or two-hand hold.

Start with feet apart, weight on right foot
1 Release hold with right hand, turn ¼ to right, left foot forward, keeping right foot in place, then release hold with left hand (2)
2 Turn ½ to right, then replace weight forward on to right foot (3)
3 Turn ¼ to right to face lady, take two-hand hold, then left foot side (small step) (4)
4 Right foot closes to left foot (&)
5 Left foot side (1)
6 Press left hand gently towards lady then release hold with left hand, turn ¼ to left, then right foot forward, keeping left foot in place and release hold with right hand (2)
7 Turn ½ to left, then replace weight forward on to left foot (3)
8 Turn ¼ to left to face lady, take closed hold or two-hand hold, then right foot side (small step) (4)
9 Left foot closes to right foot (&)
10 Right foot side (1)
End with weight on right foot
(Ball-Flat on all steps)

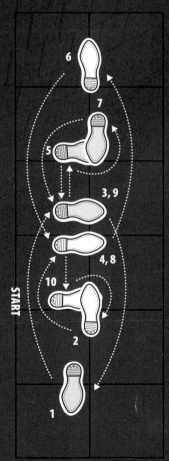

SPOT TURNS
LADY'S STEPS

Start with feet apart, weight on left foot
1 Turn ¼ to left, then right foot forward, keeping left foot in place (2)
2 Turn ½ to left, then replace weight forward on to left foot (3)
3 Turn ¼ to left to face man, then right foot side (small step) (4)
4 Left foot closes to right foot (&)
5 Right foot side (1)
6 Press right hand gently towards man, turn ¼ to right, then left foot forward, keeping right foot in place (2)
7 Turn ½ to right, then replace weight forward on to right foot (3)
8 Turn ¼ to right to face man, then left foot side (small step) (4)
9 Right foot closes to left foot (&)
10 Left foot side (1)
End with weight on left foot
(Ball-Flat on all steps)

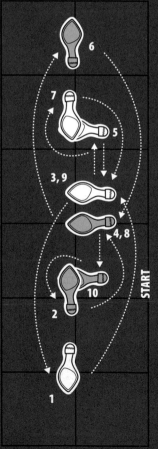

TIME STEP
MAN'S STEPS

This figure is danced without hold, facing partner.

Start with weight on right foot
1 Left foot crosses behind right foot (2)
2 Replace weight forward on to right foot (3)
3 Left foot side (small step) (4)
4 Right foot closes to left foot (&)
5 Left foot side (1)
6 Right foot crosses behind left foot (2)
7 Replace weight forward on to left foot (3)
8 Right foot side (small step) (4)
9 Left foot closes to right foot (&)
10 Right foot side (1)
End with weight on right foot
(1. & 6. Ball; all other steps Ball-Flat)

Note
Time Step may be repeated.

Resume closed hold or two-hand hold on steps 8–10 to prepare
for next figure.

TIME STEP
LADY'S STEPS

Start with weight on left foot
1 Right foot crosses behind left foot (2)
2 Replace weight forward on to left foot (3)
3 Right foot side (small step) (4)
4 Left foot closes to right foot (&)
5 Right foot side (1)
6 Left foot crosses behind right foot (2)
7 Replace weight forward on to right foot (3)
8 Left foot side (small step) (4)
9 Right foot closes to left foot (&)
10 Left foot side (1)
End with weight on left foot
(1. & 6. Ball; all other steps Ball-Flat)

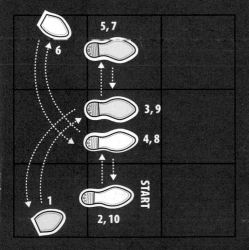

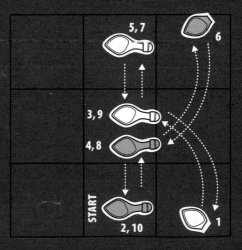

Foxtrot

The Foxtrot danced on *Strictly* is the Slow Foxtrot, which evokes the sophistication of the dance floors of the 1930s. Based on Harry Fox's 1914 dance creation, the Foxtrot is comprised of complex, technical footwork, straight-line figures, difficult heel turns and expansive poses. Its cousin, the Rhythm Foxtrot, uses slightly faster music, and has an easy-to-master slow-slow-quick-quick rhythm that makes it a classic social dance, often seen at weddings. But the more challenging Slow Foxtrot, with its slow-quick-quick rhythm and gliding movement, has become the epitome of grace and style on both the social and competition dance floors.

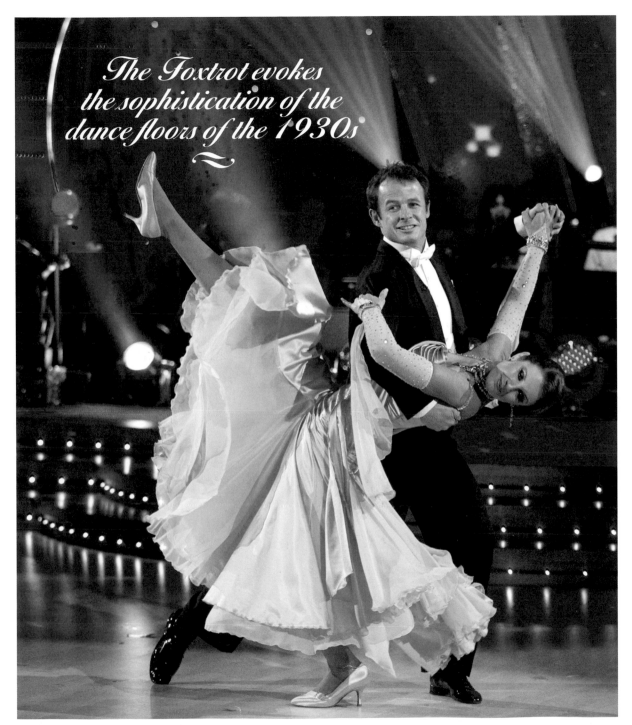

The Foxtrot evokes the sophistication of the dance floors of the 1930s

The Dance

OVERSWAY INTO AERIAL RONDÉ
The man leads the woman into an Oversway before turning and lifting her, causing her leg to swing up and to the side.

SAME-FOOT LUNGE
The couple's legs mirror each other throughout the Foxtrot, but here the dancers take their weight on to the same leg, with the free leg pointing out in the same direction, extending the line.

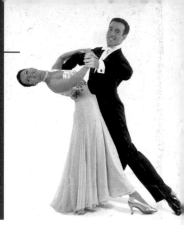

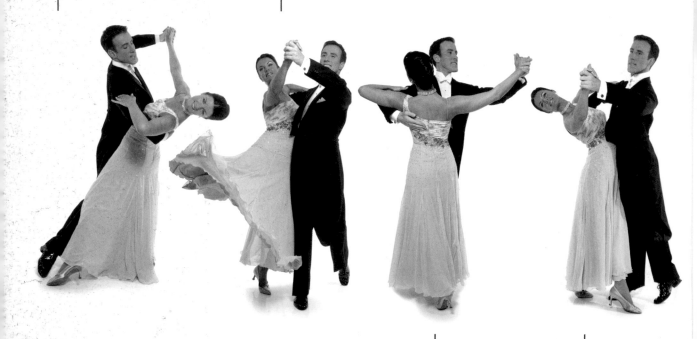

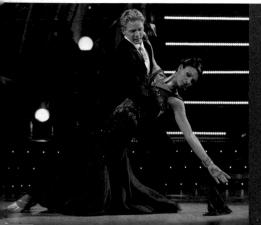

FEATHER STEP
The Feather Step, named for its original curving shape, is half the basic pattern of the Foxtrot. On step three, the man steps forward just outside the woman's right hip.

HOVER CROSS
The man steps diagonally forward outside the woman's left hip, maintaining body contact. This 'checking action' is often danced in a corner and may be followed by a Three Step.

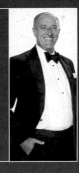

The Rumba is my favourite Latin dance, and the Foxtrot is my favourite in the ballroom section. It's one of the first ones I mastered when my girlfriend took me to dance lessons all those years ago. It's got grace and style and elegance, and, when you do it properly, you really should look as if you're dancing on air. But, in technical terms, it's a hard one. The basic step pattern is easy enough, but then you have to work so much at developing it. When we see a couple Foxtrotting, we're looking for a light, carefree attitude, as if they hardly know that they're dancing.

Foxtrot should have a smooth quality, where the body seems to be gliding across the floor while the feet dance the classic 'slow-quick-quick' rhythm underneath.

TIMING

Foxtrot music is written as '1234', with one strong beat and three weak beats, but the music may sound more like 'strong-weak, strong-weak', with the first beat being the strongest. As with all the four-beat ballroom dances, a 'slow' is one step taken at the beginning of two beats of music, and a 'quick' is a step taken over one beat of music.

MUSIC

'More' and 'Let's Fall in Love', both by Nat 'King' Cole, are Foxtrot classics. 'Mandy' (Barry Manilow) is a modern track with the requisite smooth texture. Timing is 29–30 bars per minute.

HOLD & POSTURE

The classic ballroom hold is maintained throughout the Foxtrot. The man must use his body to communicate the lead to his partner, including rise and fall, direction and amount of turn.

LEGS & FEET

A good Foxtrot has subtle rise and controlled lowering. Toes should release from the floor in backward walks. Precise heel turns in Natural and Reverse Turns get high marks from the judges.

DRESS

As with the Waltz, the man is in ballroom tails, and the woman's dress is elegant and flowing. Pastel colours emphasize the soft, floating quality of the dance.

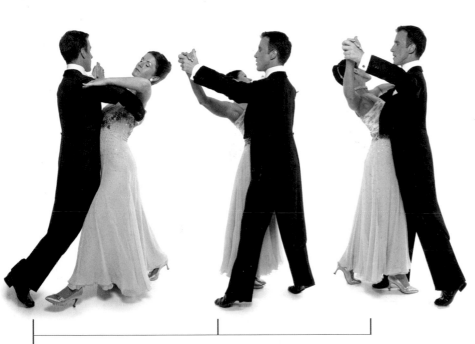

HEEL TURNS

In this Reverse Turn sequence (to the left), Anton takes the second step sideways in front of Erin, causing her to pivot on her heel. They then step out of the turn together.

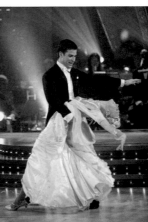

The Steps

FEATHER STEP
MAN'S STEPS

This figure is danced in closed hold.

Start with weight on left foot
1 Right foot forward (S)
2 Left foot forward (left side leading) (Q)
3 Right foot forward outside partner (Q)
End with weight on right foot
(1. Heel-Toe, 2. Toe, 3. Toe-Heel)

FEATHER STEP
LADY'S STEPS

Start with weight on right foot
1 Left foot back (S)
2 Right foot back (Q)
3 Left foot back (Q)
End with weight on left foot
(1. Toe-Heel, 2. Toe-Heel, 3. Toe-Heel)

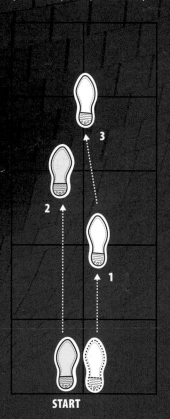

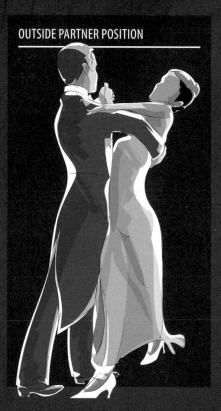

OUTSIDE PARTNER POSITION

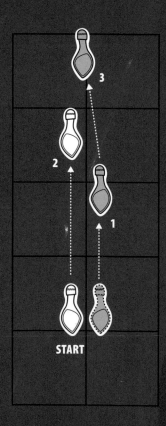

THREE STEP
MAN'S STEPS

This figure is danced in closed hold.

Start with weight forward on right foot outside partner
1 Left foot forward (S)
2 Right foot forward (Q)
3 Left foot forward (Q)
End with weight on left foot
(1. Heel, 2. Heel-Toe, 3. Toe-Heel)

THREE STEP
LADY'S STEPS

Start with weight back on left foot
1 Right foot back (S)
2 Left foot back (Q)
3 Right foot back (Q)
End with weight on right foot
(1. Toe-Heel, 2. Toe-Heel, 3. Toe-Heel)

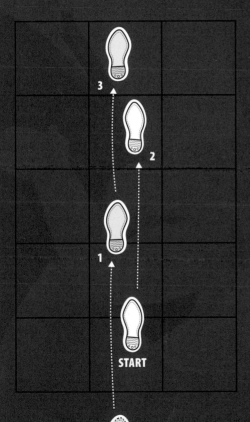

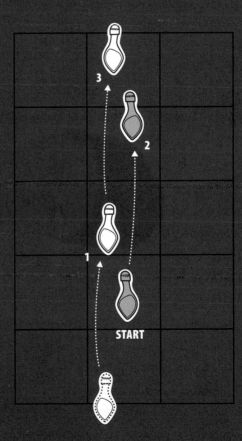

The Steps

NATURAL TURN
MAN'S STEPS

This figure is danced in closed hold.

Start with weight on left foot

1 Right foot forward, starting to turn to right (S)

2 Turn ⅜ to right, then left foot side (Q)

3 Turn ⅛ to right, then right foot back (Q)

4 Left foot back, starting to turn to right (S)

5 Turn ¼ to right, then right foot side (small step) (S)

6 Left foot forward (S)

End with weight on left foot

(1. Heel-Toe, 2. Toe, 3. Toe-Heel, 4. Toe-Heel, 5. Heel-Whole foot, 6. Heel-Flat)

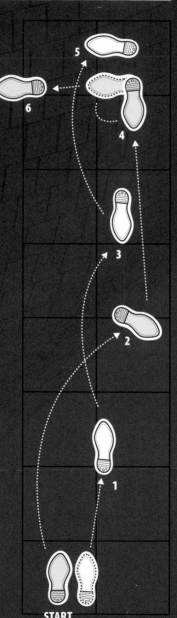

NATURAL TURN
LADY'S STEPS

Start with weight on right foot

1 Left foot back (S)

2 On heel of left foot, turn ½ to right ('heel turn'), then right foot closes to left foot (Q)

3 Left foot forward (Q)

4 Right foot forward (S)

5 Turn ¼ to right, then left foot side (S)

6 Right foot back (S)

End with weight on right foot

(1. Toe-Heel, 2. Heel-Toe, 3. Toe-Heel, 4. Heel, 5. Toe-Whole foot, 6. Toe-Flat)

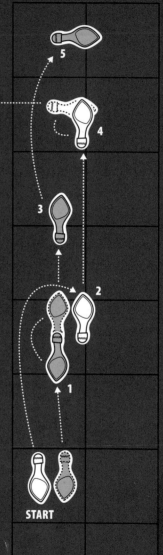

CHANGE OF DIRECTION
MAN'S STEPS

This figure is danced in closed hold.

Start with weight forward on right foot outside partner
1 Left foot forward (S)
2 Right foot forward, then turn ¼ to left (S)
3 Left foot forward (S)
End with weight on left foot
(1. Heel, 2. Toe-Whole foot, 3. Heel-Flat)

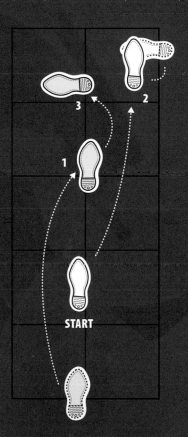

CHANGE OF DIRECTION
LADY'S STEPS

Start with weight back on left foot
1 Right foot back (S)
2 Left foot back, then turn ¼ to left (S)
3 Right foot back (S)
End with weight on right foot
(1. Toe-Heel, 2. Toe-Whole foot,
3. Toe-Flat)

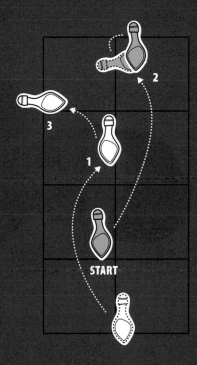

SUGGESTED AMALGAMATIONS

Feather Step – Three Step (repeat both figures, dancing
    them around the room)
Feather Step – Change of Direction (in corner)
Three Step – Natural Turn (in corner)

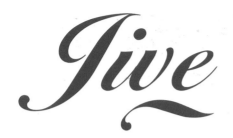

Jive

The Jive is the lightest and brightest of the Latin American dances, allowing the dancers to express pure joy, playfulness and fun. The first recognized form of Jive, the Lindy Hop, came about in the jazz-crazed 1920s. Then American GIs brought a new form of the dance, the Jitterbug, to Europe in the 1940s, where it was considered a 'corrupting influence' (just like the Waltz had been over a hundred years earlier). During the 1950s, the dance mutated into Swing, Boogie-Woogie and Rock'n'Roll. What we now call Jive includes elements of these previous forms, but continues to evolve as dancers explore its exuberant choreography.

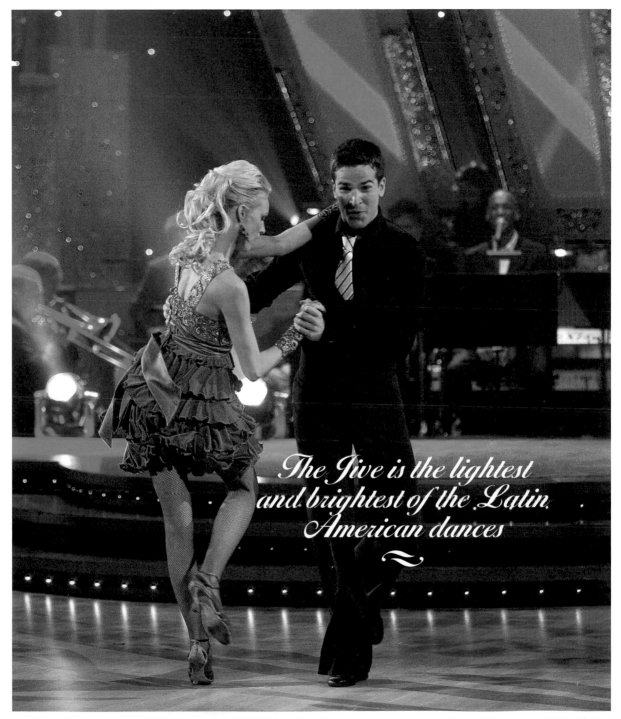

The Jive is the lightest and brightest of the Latin American dances

The Dance

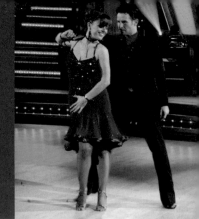

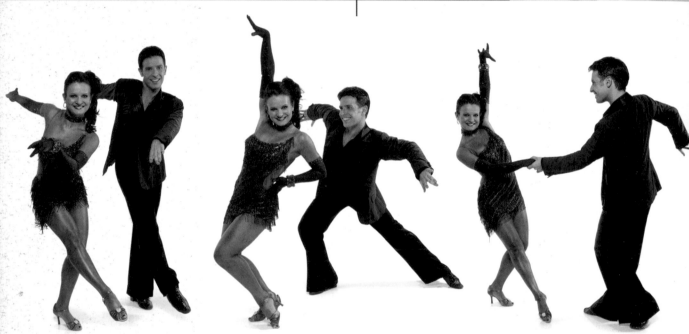

KICKS AND FLICKS
Kicks are made from the hip joint, and flicks are made from the knee. Sharp flicks with pointed toes get good marks from the judges.

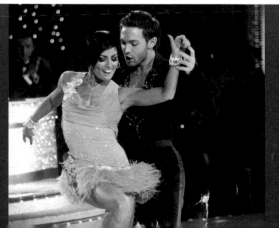

CHICKEN WALKS
A classic Jive step, in which the man dances a strong hip action as he guides the woman towards him. Lilia swivels from foot to foot while Darren supports her.

LEN'S OVERVIEW

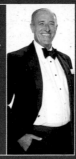

The Jive should be a bright and lively dance, a mixture of many different styles, so we're always looking for inventive choreography. But you have to have technique as well, otherwise you end up like some of the contestants on the show — just running around the floor waving their hands in the air and doing no footwork at all. Jive can look pretty free-form at times, but, in fact, it's a stylized dance that takes elements from all over the place — and you'd better get them right or it's going to be a mess.

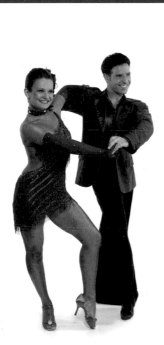

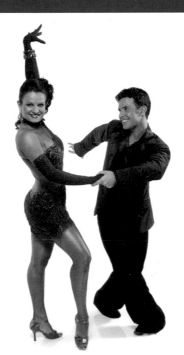

BACK ROCK

The Back Rock is included in almost every Jive figure. Starting in closed hold, the dancers turn away from each other, step back, then replace their weight forward.

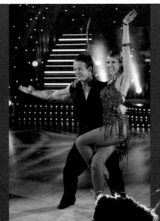

STOP AND GO

The couple dances the beginning of a Change of Place Left to Right, followed by a checking action, and finishing with the beginning of a Change of Place Right to Left.

Jive should be danced with a playful bounce in the knees, making this a good dance for leg and cardiovascular fitness. Swinging the hips from side to side keeps the waist trim!

TIMING

The musical rhythm is '1234', with the first beat as the strongest. The figures are danced over six beats of music. There are 'a' beats interspersed between strong and weak beats. Steps 4 and 7 are danced on 'a' beats.

MUSIC

There is great Jive music for every dancer's taste, including 'Boogie-Woogie Bugle Boy' by The Andrew Sisters, 'Crazy Little Thing Called Love' by Queen, 'Blue Suede Shoes' by Elvis Presley and 'Candyman' by Christina Aguilera. Jive is played at 42–44 bars per minute.

HOLD & POSTURE

Jive posture is quite upright, although, for Lindy Hop moves, dancers can bend forward at the hips. Toned arms must connect with the partner and hit clear lines. No floppy fingers, please!

LEGS & FEET

Small, quick flicks of the lower leg are quintessentially Jive. Clever footwork is the name of the game, and all movements should be precise and complete.

DRESS

The Jive wardrobe has eclectic roots. Darren's wearing a 50s-style purple jacket — very rock'n'roll — while Lilia's matching dress with its bead fringing is redolent of the 1920s and 30s.

The Steps

BASIC STEP
MAN'S STEPS

This figure is danced in closed hold.

Start with weight on right foot
1 Turn slightly to left, then left foot back (1)
2 Replace weight forward on to right foot (2)
3 Turn slightly to right to face lady, then left foot side (small step) (3)
4 Right foot closes towards left foot (a)
5 Left foot side (4)
6 Right foot side (small step) (5)
7 Left foot closes towards right foot (a)
8 Right foot side (6)
End with weight on right foot
(1. Ball-Flat, 2. Ball-Flat, 3. Ball, 4. Whole foot, 5. Ball-Flat, 6. Ball, 7. Whole foot, 8. Ball-Flat)

Note
If preceding figure ends in single-hand hold, then resume closed hold over steps 3–5 of Basic Step.

BASIC STEP
LADY'S STEPS

Start with weight on left foot
1 Turn up to ¼ to right, then right foot back (1)
2 Replace weight forward on to left foot (2)
3 Turn ¼ to left to face man, then right foot side (small step) (3)
4 Left foot closes towards right foot (a)
5 Right foot side (4)
6 Left foot side (small step) (5)
7 Right foot closes towards left foot (a)
8 Left foot side (6)
End with weight on left foot
(1. Ball-Flat, 2. Ball-Flat, 3. Ball, 4. Whole foot, 5. Ball-Flat, 6. Ball, 7. Whole foot, 8. Ball-Flat)

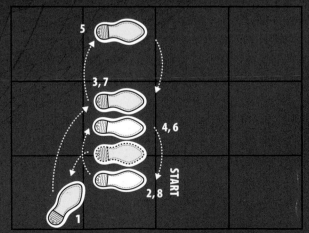

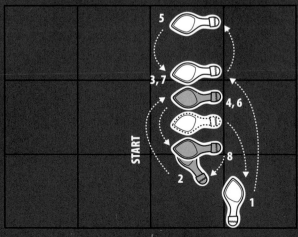

CHANGE OF PLACE RIGHT TO LEFT
MAN'S STEPS

This figure starts in closed hold and ends in single-hand hold.

Start with weight on right foot
1 Turn slightly to left, then left foot back (1)
2 Replace weight forward on to right foot (2)
3 Left foot side (small step), and lift left hand near left shoulder to prepare lady to turn (3)
4 Right foot closes towards left foot (a)
5 Left foot side, and lift left hand over lady's head, turning her clockwise over steps 6–8 (4)
6 Right foot side (small step), starting to turn to left (5)
7 Continuing to turn to left, left foot closes towards right foot (a)
8 Right foot side facing lady, and relax left arm down, having turned ¼ to left over steps 6–8 (6)
End with weight on right foot
(1. Ball-Flat, 2. Ball-Flat, 3. Ball, 4. Whole foot, 5. Ball-Flat, 6. Ball, 7. Whole foot, 8. Ball-Flat)

CHANGE OF PLACE RIGHT TO LEFT
LADY'S STEPS

Start with weight on left foot
1 Turn ¼ to right, then right foot back (1)
2 Replace weight forward on to left foot (2)
3 Turn ¼ to left to face man, then right foot side (small step) (3)
4 Left foot closes towards right foot (a)
5 Right foot side, then ½ turn to right under raised right arm (4)
6 Continue to turn to right, then left foot side (small step) (5)
7 Continue to turn to right, right foot closes towards left foot (a)
8 Left foot side facing man, having turned ¼ to right over steps 6–8 (6)
End with weight on left foot
(1. Ball-Flat, 2. Ball-Flat, 3. Ball, 4. Whole foot, 5. Ball-Flat, 6. Ball, 7. Whole foot, 8. Ball-Flat)

Note
Lady turns a total of ¾ to right over steps 5–8.

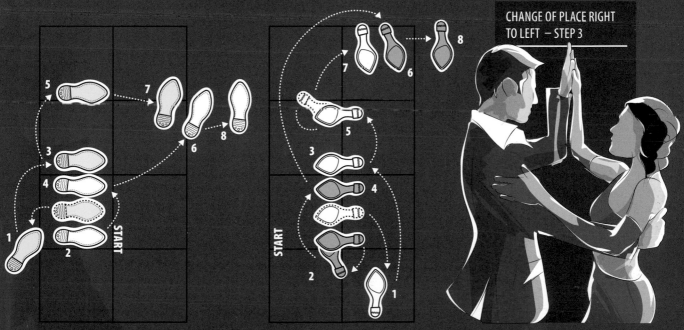

CHANGE OF PLACE RIGHT TO LEFT – STEP 3

The Steps

CHANGE OF PLACE LEFT TO RIGHT
MAN'S STEPS

This figure starts and ends in single-hand hold.

Start with weight on right foot
1 Left foot back (1)
2 Replace weight forward on to right foot (2)
3 Left foot side (small step), starting to turn to right, and lift left arm (3)
4 Continuing to turn to right, right foot closes towards left foot (a)
5 Left foot side, having turned ¼ to right to face lady and looping left hand anticlockwise over lady's head (4)
6 Right foot side (5)
7 Left foot closes towards right foot (a)
8 Right foot side, and relax left arm down when lady completes turn (6)
End with weight on right foot
(1. Ball-Flat, 2. Ball-Flat, 3. Ball, 4. Whole foot, 5. Ball-Flat, 6. Ball, 7. Whole foot, 8. Ball-Flat)

CHANGE OF PLACE LEFT TO RIGHT
LADY'S STEPS

Start with weight on left foot
1 Right foot back (1)
2 Replace weight forward on to left foot (2)
3 Turn ¼ to left, then right foot side (small step) (3)
4 Left foot closes towards right foot (a)
5 Right foot side, then turn ½ to left to face man (4)
6 Left foot side (small step) (5)
7 Right foot closes towards left foot (a)
8 Left foot side (6)
End with weight on left foot
(1. Ball-Flat, 2. Ball-Flat, 3. Ball, 4. Whole foot, 5. Ball-Flat, 6. Ball, 7. Whole foot, 8. Ball-Flat)

Note
Lady turns a total of ¾ to left over steps 5–8.

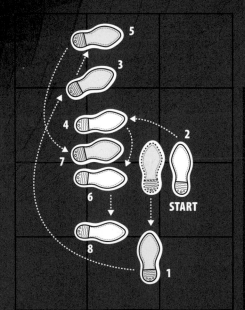

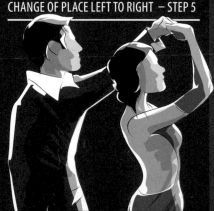

CHANGE OF PLACE LEFT TO RIGHT – STEP 5

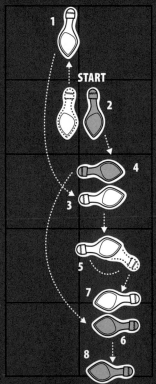

AMERICAN SPIN
MAN'S STEPS

This figure starts and ends in single-hand hold.

Start with weight on right foot
1 Left foot back (1)
2 Replace weight forward on to right foot (2)
3 Left foot closes to right foot, and brace left arm over steps 3–5 to bring lady close (3)
4 Right foot steps in place (a)
5 Left foot steps in place – then with left arm give gentle push forward to lead lady to spin, and release lady (4)
6 Right foot steps in place (5)
7 Left foot steps in place (a)
8 Right foot steps in place – with left hand take hold of lady's right hand when she finishes turning (6)
End with weight on right foot

AMERICAN SPIN
LADY'S STEPS

Start with weight on left foot
1 Right foot back (1)
2 Replace weight forward on to left foot (2)
3 Right foot forward (small step) (3)
4 Left foot closes towards right foot (a)
5 Right foot forward (small step) – then, with right arm, gently push away from man and turn ¾ to right (4)
6 Continue to turn to right, then left foot side (small step) (5)
7 Continue to turn to right, then right foot closes towards left foot (a)
8 Left foot side facing man, having turned ¼ turn to right over steps 6–8 (6)
End with weight on left foot
(For both man's and lady's steps: 1. Ball-Flat, 2. Ball-Flat, 3. Ball, 4. Whole foot, 5. Ball-Flat, 6. Ball, 7. Whole foot, 8. Ball-Flat)

Note
Lady turns a total of one full turn over steps 5–8.

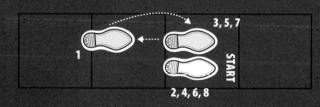

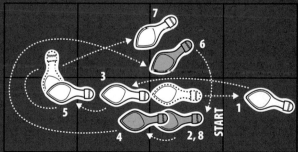

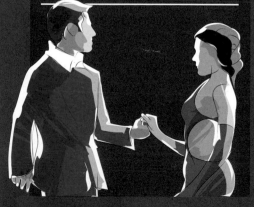

SINGLE-HAND HOLD

SUGGESTED AMALGAMATIONS

Basic Step – Change of Place Right to Left – Change of Place Left to Right

Basic Step – Change of Place Right to Left – Change of Place Left to Right – American Spin (once or twice)

Paso Doble

The ultimate expression of dance machismo, in the Paso Doble the man plays the role of the fearless Spanish matador, while the woman plays both the cape and the bull. This dance, one of the biggest challenges for the *Strictly Come Dancing* contestants, is a stylized representation of the Spanish bullfight (*corrida*). It's a deadly serious dance, charged with drama, passion and violence. Based on the marching music at the beginning of the bullfight, the Paso Doble developed into a popular social dance in France in the 1930s. Today, the Paso Doble is the most dramatic and narrative of the competitive Latin American dances.

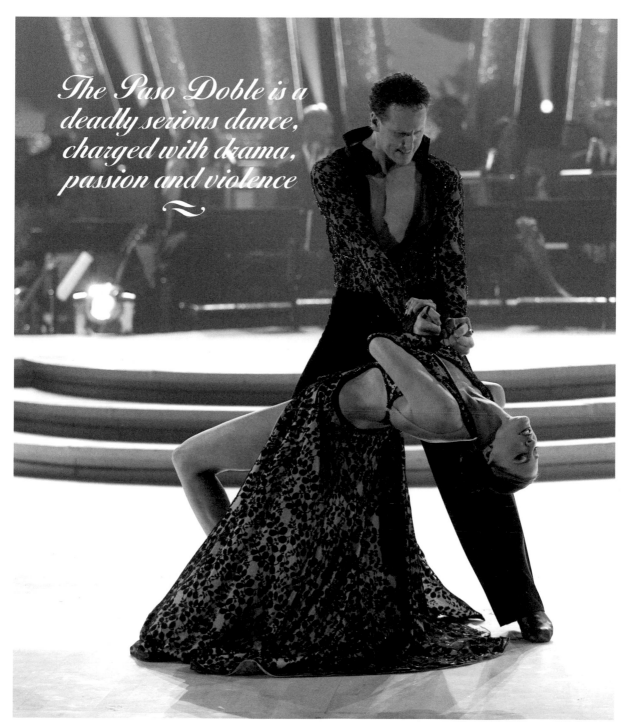

The Paso Doble is a deadly serious dance, charged with drama, passion and violence

The Dance

CHASSÉ CAPE

The man passes the woman in front of him, imitating the bullfighter passing the cape as the bull charges past. A strong hold is essential to maintain balance.

COUP DE PIQUE

Pointed toes represent the swords stabbing the bull to death. It's important that the dancers have serious expressions throughout the Paso Doble, especially at these dramatic moments.

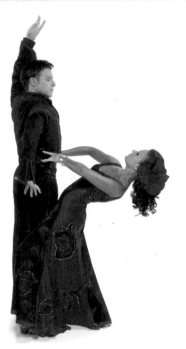

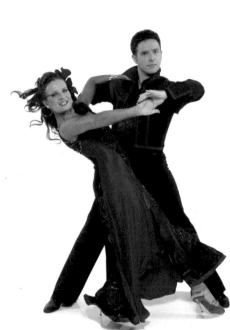

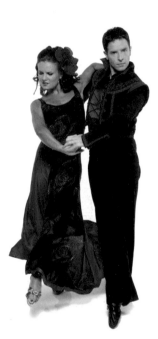

MALE DOMINANCE

As the bullfighter, the man should accentuate his mastery of the situation by his movements. In this posture, the woman bowing backwards represents the man's cape.

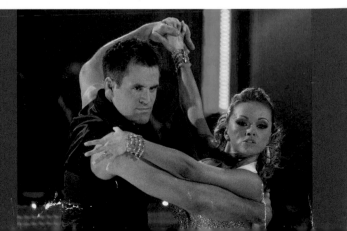

You have to take this dance seriously and do it with commitment, otherwise it's not worth bothering. I look for good posture from the man, toned to the tips of his fingers, and for big, dramatic shapes from the woman. And they must look the part. It's no good going into a Paso Doble with a big smile. I want to see them looking angry — aggressive even. Their eyes should always be focused, either on each other, on a judge, or even on a member of the audience. They must maintain that intensity right through the dance.

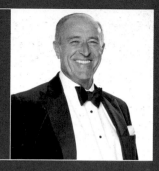

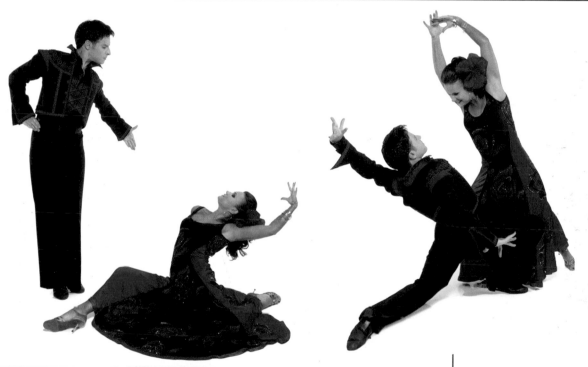

MATADOR THROWS CAPE
The bullfighter tosses the cape disdainfully to the ground. Lilia uses her skirt to represent the cape's cloth, while Darren shows the erect line of the bullfighter.

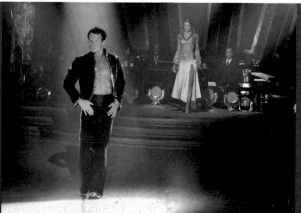

ROLE REVERSAL
Sometimes the bull gets the upper hand — but the bullfighter shows who's in charge by dropping down to demonstrate that he isn't impressed.

SIDE STEPS

A bit of all-important basic, Side Steps are a series of small steps that can be danced to the left or right with flexed knees or up on the toes.

TWIST TURNS

Once again, the woman is the cape being worked by the bullfighter. She curves around in front of him as he turns on the balls of his feet.

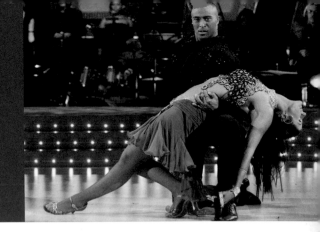

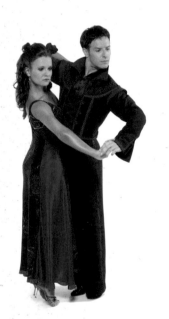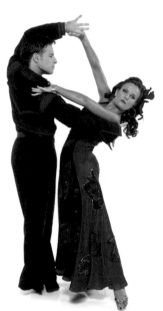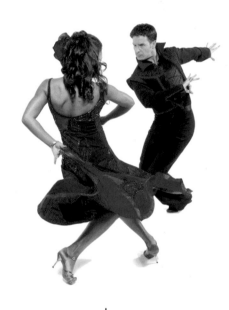

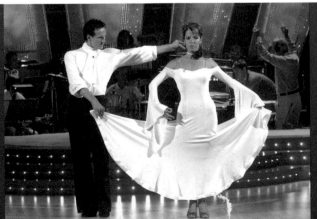

FLAMENCO CHECKS

The couple dance in front of each other in a series of flexed-leg movements going from right to left, building up intensity in the battle for dominance.

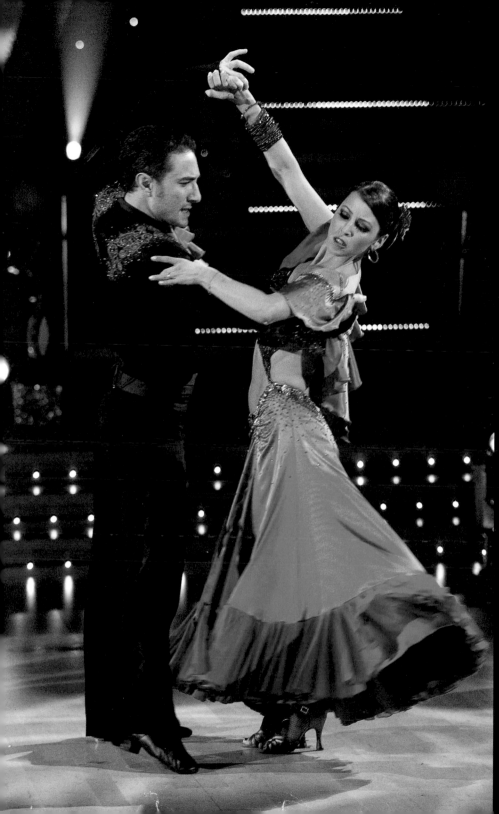

Paso Doble is about danger and drama. The dance requires a flexible spine, strong legs and good core strength to perform the exaggerated movements and shapes of the dance.

TIMING

Paso Doble music has one strong and one weak beat, but both beats feel equal in strength, giving the movement a marching quality. The steps in this book start on the first strong beat. There are also 'highlights' in the music that dancers punctuate with theatrical shapes and lines to give a dramatic effect.

MUSIC

'Spanish Gypsy Dance' is the most recognizable music. 'Y Viva España' and 'L'España Cañi' are also popular, and all are written in 2/4 'march' style, played at 60 bars per minute.

HOLD & POSTURE

Large movements are created by shaping through the spine. Arms and hands with flamenco styling express strength in the man and suppleness in the woman.

LEGS & FEET

Leg strength is required to perform the lunges and leaps. Toned feet are used as a storytelling device: to attract the bull's attention, or to represent the sword. Flamenco rhythmic stamping can be used to decorate the dance.

DRESS

Darren wears a stylized version of a bullfighter's bolero, black trimmed in red, while Lilia picks up the same colours in a flamenco-styled outfit with a tight bodice and full skirt. Natasha Kaplinsky's white dress (see opposite page) had a full skirt that doubled as the cape.

The Steps

SUR PLACE
MAN'S STEPS

This figure is danced in closed hold. Sur Place may be danced turning to the left or right.

Start with weight on left foot
1 Right foot in place (1)
2 Left foot in place (2)
3 Right foot in place (3)
4 Left foot in place (4)
5 Right foot in place (5)
6 Left foot in place (6)
7 Right foot in place (7)
8 Left foot in place (8)
End with weight on left foot
(Ball on all steps)

Note
Sur Place may turn to left or right.

SUR PLACE
LADY'S STEPS

Start with weight on right foot
1 Left foot in place (1)
2 Right foot in place (2)
3 Left foot in place (3)
4 Right foot in place (4)
5 Left foot in place (5)
6 Right foot in place (6)
7 Left foot in place (7)
8 Right foot in place (8)
End with weight on right foot
(Ball on all steps)

SEPARATIONS
MAN'S STEPS

This figure starts and ends in closed hold.

Start with weight on left foot
1 Right foot in place (1)
2 Left foot forward (2)
3 Release hold with right arm,
then right foot closes to
left foot (3)
4 Left foot in place (4)
5 Right foot in place (5)
6 Left foot in place (6)
7 Right foot in place (7)
8 Left foot in place (8)
End with weight on left foot
(1. Whole foot, 2. Heel, 3. Ball,
4. Ball, 5. Ball, 6. Ball, 7. Ball,
8. Ball-Flat)

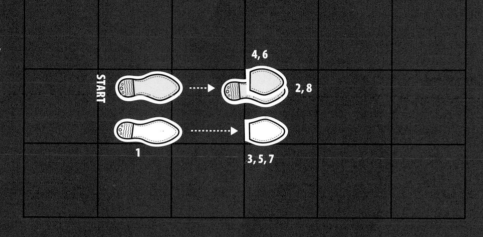

SEPARATIONS
LADY'S STEPS

Start with weight on right foot
1 Left foot in place (1)
2 Right foot back (2)
3 Left foot back (3)
4 Right foot closes to left
foot (4)
5 Left foot forward (5)
6 Right foot forward (6)
7 Left foot forward (7)
8 Right foot forward (8)
End with weight on right foot
(1. Whole foot, 2. Ball-Flat,
3. Ball, 4. Ball, 5. Ball, 6. Ball,
7. Ball, 8. Ball-Flat)

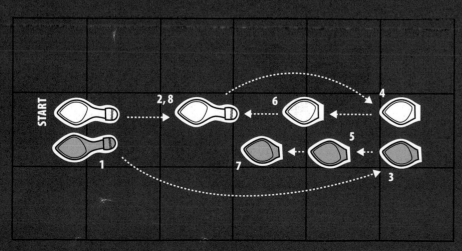

The Steps

PROMENADE
MAN'S STEPS

This figure is danced in closed hold.

Start with weight on left foot
1 Turn ⅛ to left to promenade position, then right foot in place (1)
2 Left foot side in promenade position (2)
3 Right foot forward and across in promenade position (3)
4 Turn ⅜ to right, then left foot diagonally back (4)
5 Right foot back (5)
6 Left foot back (6)
7 Turn ¼ to right, then right foot side (7)
8 Left foot closes to right foot (8)
End with weight on left foot
(1. Whole foot, 2. Heel-Flat, 3. Heel-Flat, 4. Ball-Flat, 5. Ball-Flat, 6. Ball-Flat, 7.Ball, 8. Ball)

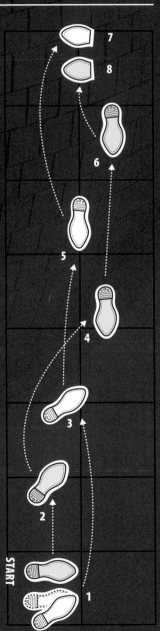

PROMENADE
LADY'S STEPS

Start with weight on right foot
1 Turn ⅛ to right to promenade position, then left foot in place (1)
2 Right foot side in promenade position (2)
3 Left foot forward and across in promenade position (3)
4 Turn ⅛ to right, then right foot forward (4)
5 Left foot forward (5)
6 Right foot forward outside partner (6)
7 Turn ¼ to right, then left foot side (7)
8 Right foot closes to left foot (8)
End with weight on right foot
(1. Whole foot, 2. Heel-Flat, 3. Heel-Flat, 4. Heel-Flat, 5. Heel-Flat, 6. Heel-Flat, 7. Ball, 8. Ball)

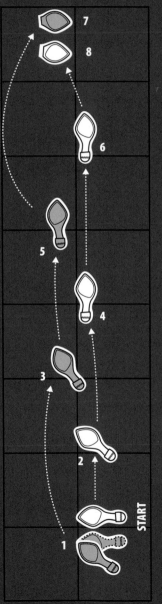

COUP DE PIQUE
MAN'S STEPS

This figure starts and ends in closed hold.

Start with weight on left foot
1 Turn ⅛ to left to promenade position, then point right foot forward without weight (1)
2 Turn ⅛ to right to closed hold, then right foot closes to left foot (2)
3 Turn ⅛ to left to promenade position, then left foot back (3)
4 Turn ⅛ to right to closed hold, then right foot closes to left foot (4)
5 Turn ⅛ to left to promenade position, then left foot back (5)
6 Turn ⅛ to right to closed hold, then right foot side (6)
7 Left foot closes to right foot (&)
8 Right foot side (7)
9 Left foot closes to right foot (8)

End with weight on left foot
(1. Point toe; all other steps Ball)

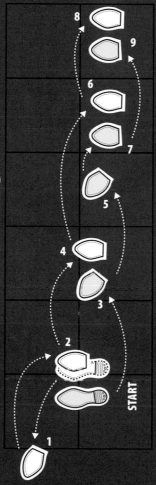

COUP DE PIQUE
LADY'S STEPS

Start with weight on right foot
1 Turn ⅛ to right to promenade position, then point left foot forward without weight (1)
2 Turn ⅛ to left to closed hold, then left foot closes to right foot (2)
3 Turn ⅛ to right to promenade position, then right foot back (3)
4 Turn ⅛ to left to closed hold, then left foot closes to right foot (4)
5 Turn ⅛ to right to promenade position, then right foot back (5)
6 Turn ⅛ to left to closed hold, then left foot side (6)
7 Right foot closes to left foot (&)
8 Left foot side (7)
9 Right foot closes to left foot (8)

End with weight on right foot
(1. Point toe; all other steps Ball)

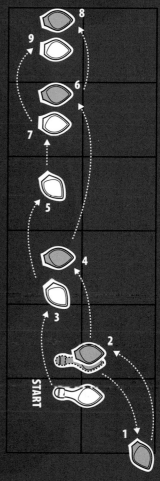

SUGGESTED AMALGAMATIONS

Sur Place – Separations
Sur Place – Promenade – Sur Place turning ½ either to left or right
Sur Place – Promenade – Separations – Coup de Pique – Sur Place turning ½ either to left or right

Quickstep

The Quickstep, the happiest of the ballroom dances, gives the ballroom brigade a chance to show off some pretty fancy footwork. This vibrant dance takes the couple speeding around the floor in a mixture of classic gliding movements, Charleston kicks and more hops than the Easter Bunny. As the Foxtrot became the most popular dance of the 1920s, bands started to play the music faster, making it hard for all but the most skilful couples to keep up with them. So the Quickstep was born and, with its myriad syncopated steps, hops, skips and spins, it has become a dynamic dance of seemingly endless possibilities.

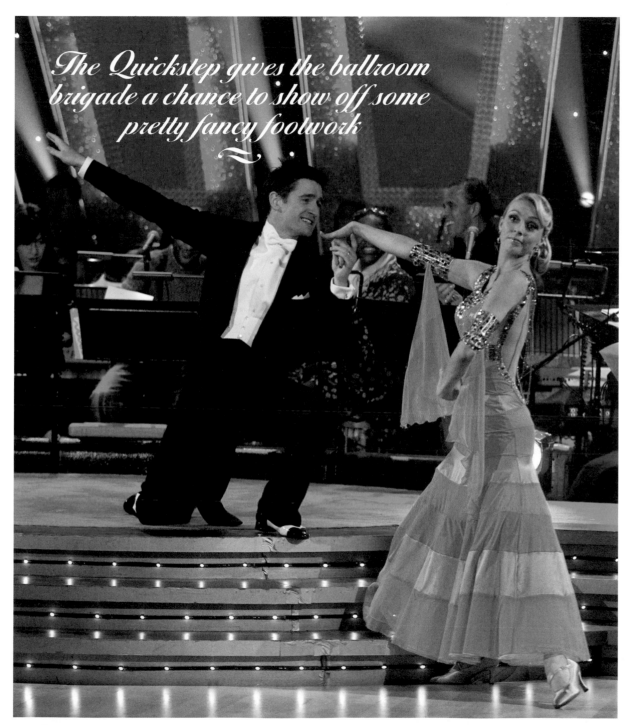

The Quickstep gives the ballroom brigade a chance to show off some pretty fancy footwork

The Dance

LOCKSTEP

One of the most basic elements of the Quickstep. One foot crosses behind or in front of the other, showing the dancer's alacrity and fleetness of foot.

SPIN TURN

A rotational action often performed at the corners of the dance floor. This classic figure is used in Waltz as well and, done correctly, it makes the woman's skirt float and twist.

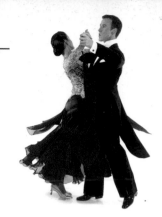

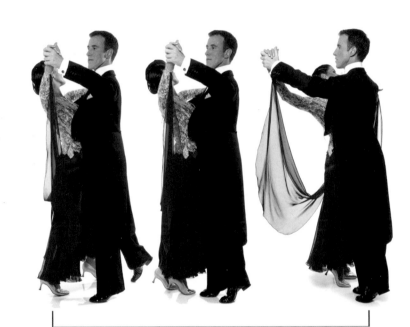

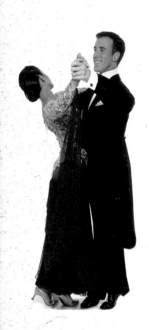

CHARLESTON

An element of the 1920s dance craze with many variations. Here, Anton and Erin show the characteristic upwards flick of the foot.

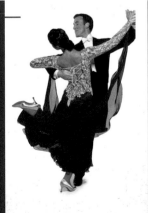

LOCKSTEP SEQUENCE

The Lockstep can be danced both forward and backward. Here Anton goes forward on to his left foot, Erin steps back on to her right, and they both cross their feet with the other foot.

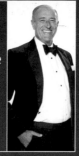

LEN'S OVERVIEW

The Quickstep is all about the mood. It's actually quite a simple dance, and there aren't that many steps, so the dancers have to score points by getting the right mixture of smooth, gliding action and fast, showy kicks and flicks. When a Quickstep is done well, you should be watching it with a big grin on your face because it's so light and joyful. Anton and Erin are so light they're almost floating away.

Quickstep, the fastest of the ballroom dances, provides a good cardiovascular workout thanks to all the skips and hops. Even Olympic champion Denise Lewis was left breathless by this dance.

TIMING
Quickstep is one of the '1234' dances with a heavy first beat and three light beats, but the rhythm is 'heavy-light, heavy-light', with the third beat not quite as heavy as the first beat. Dance an amalgamation by taking the first step of the first figure on the strong '1' beat, then follow the pattern of 'quicks' and 'slows' for each figure.

MUSIC
Classic tracks such as 'Let's Face the Music and Dance' (the Nat 'King' Cole version) and 'Sing, Sing, Sing' (the Benny Goodman Orchestra) give the right feel for this speedy dance, played at 50–52 bars per minute.

HOLD & POSTURE
The ballroom hold is fundamentally the same, but it must be both firm and light: firm to hold the spinning partnership together; light to allow for the quickness of movement and changes of direction.

LEGS & FEET
Rapid weight changes from foot to foot give the Quickstep its skipping, tripping character. Feet are light on the floor with rapid brushes and pivots, giving the dancers an impression of weightlessness.

DRESS
Floating chiffon panels and a layered skirt create a whirlwind of movement around the woman's legs, giving more lift and sweep to the dance. Classic tails reinforce the elegant look of this ballroom dance.

PIVOTS
The dancers place their right legs between each other's legs as they turn continuously around. The man's tails and the woman's skirt add volume to the movement.

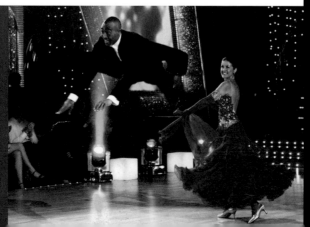

The Steps

QUARTER TURN TO RIGHT
MAN'S STEPS

This figure is danced in closed hold.

Start with weight on left foot
1 Right foot forward outside partner (S)
2 Turn ⅛ to right, then left foot side (Q)
3 Turn ⅛ to right, then right foot closes to left foot (Q)
4 Left foot side and slightly back (S)
End with weight on left foot
(1. Heel-Toe, 2. Toe, 3. Toe, 4. Toe-Heel)

QUARTER TURN TO RIGHT
LADY'S STEPS

Start with weight on right foot
1 Left foot back (S)
2 Turn ¼ to right, then right foot side (Q)
3 Left foot closes to right foot (Q)
4 Right foot side and slightly forward (S)
End with weight on right foot
(1. Toe-Heel, 2. Toe, 3. Toe, 4. Toe-Heel)

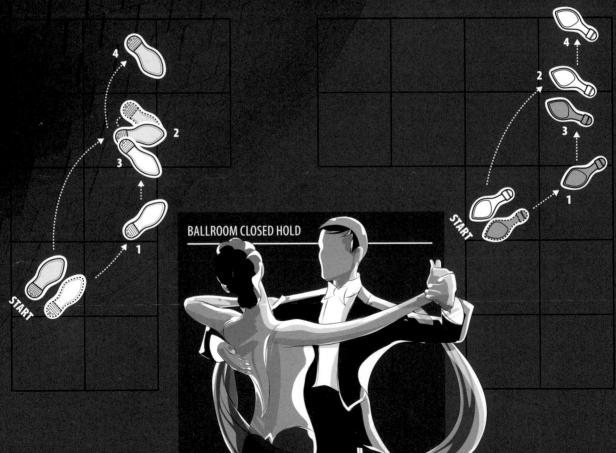

BALLROOM CLOSED HOLD

PROGRESSIVE CHASSÉ
MAN'S STEPS

This figure is danced in closed hold.

Start with weight on left foot
1 Right foot back (S)
2 Turn ¼ to left, then left foot side (Q)
3 Right foot closes to left foot (Q)
4 Left foot side and slightly forward (S)
End with weight on right foot
(1. Toe-Heel, 2. Toe, 3. Toe, 4. Toe-Heel)

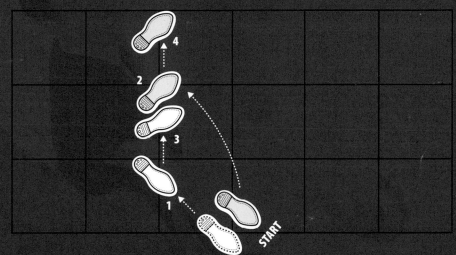

PROGRESSIVE CHASSÉ
LADY'S STEPS

Start with weight on right foot
1 Left foot forward (S)
2 Turn ⅛ to left, then right foot side (Q)
3 Turn ⅛ to left, then left foot closes to right foot (Q)
4 Right foot side and slightly back (S)
End with weight on right foot
(1. Heel-Toe, 2. Toe, 3. Toe, 4. Toe-Heel)

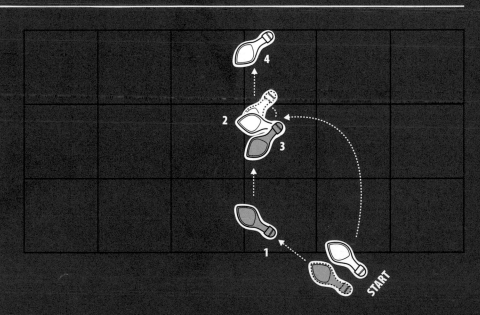

The Steps

FORWARD LOCK
MAN'S STEPS

This figure is danced in closed hold.

Start with weight on left foot
1 Right foot forward outside partner (S)
2 Left foot forward (Q)
3 Right foot crosses behind left foot (Q)
4 Left foot forward (S)
End with weight on left foot
(1. Heel-Toe, 2. Toe, 3. Toe, 4. Toe-Heel)

FORWARD LOCK
LADY'S STEPS

Start with weight on right foot
1 Left foot back (S)
2 Right foot back (Q)
3 Left foot crosses in front of right foot (Q)
4 Right foot back (S)
End with weight on right foot
(1. Toe-Heel, 2. Toe, 3. Toe, 4. Toe-Heel)

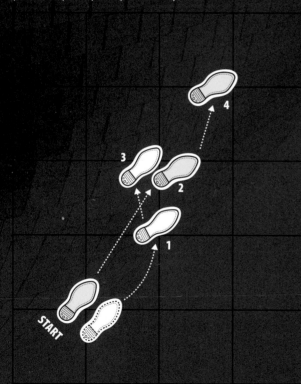

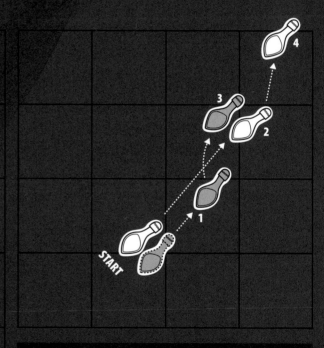

SUGGESTED AMALGAMATIONS

Quarter Turn to Right – Progressive Chassé (repeat)
Quarter Turn to Right – Progressive Chassé – Forward Lock (repeat)
Quarter Turn to Right – Progressive Chassé – Natural Turn (in corner)
Quarter Turn to Right – Progressive Chassé – Forward Lock – Natural Turn (in corner)

NATURAL TURN
MAN'S STEPS

This figure is danced in closed hold.

Start with weight on left foot
1 Right foot forward outside partner (S)
2 Turn ¼ to right, then left foot side (Q)
3 Turn ⅛ to right, then right foot closes to left foot (Q)
4 Left foot back (S)
5 Turn ⅜ to right, then right foot side (small step) (S)
6 Left foot forward (S)
End with weight on left foot
(1. Heel-Toe, 2. Toe, 3. Toe-Heel, 4. Toe-Heel, 5. Heel-Whole foot,
6. Heel-Flat)

NATURAL TURN
LADY'S STEPS

Start with weight on right foot
1 Left foot back (S)
2 Turn ⅜ to right, then right foot side (Q)
3 Left foot closes to right foot (Q)
4 Right foot forward (S)
5 Turn ¼ to right, then left foot side (S)
6 Turn ⅛ to right, then right foot back (S)
End with weight on right foot
(1. Toe-Heel, 2. Toe, 3. Toe-Heel, 4. Heel-Toe, 5. Toe-Whole foot,
6. Toe-Flat)

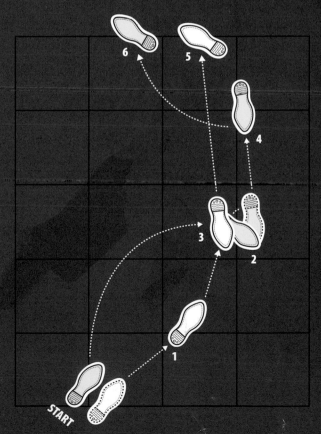

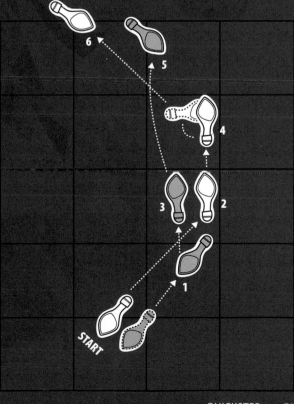

Rumba

From Africa, via Cuba and America, the Rumba burns up the dance floor with an irresistible mixture of rhythm and sexual passion. The romantic Rumba, the only slow Latin American dance, is full of enticement and seduction. The Rumba's origins are ancient, going back to African ritual dances that were transported to the New World with the slave trade. It surfaced in its modern form in Cuba in the 1890s, and was repressed by the authorities for its 'lewdness' and overt sexual overtones, but a sanitized version became popular in America in the 1930s. Because of the control required when dancing slowly, Rumba is one of the most difficult dances to master, but one of the sexiest to perform.

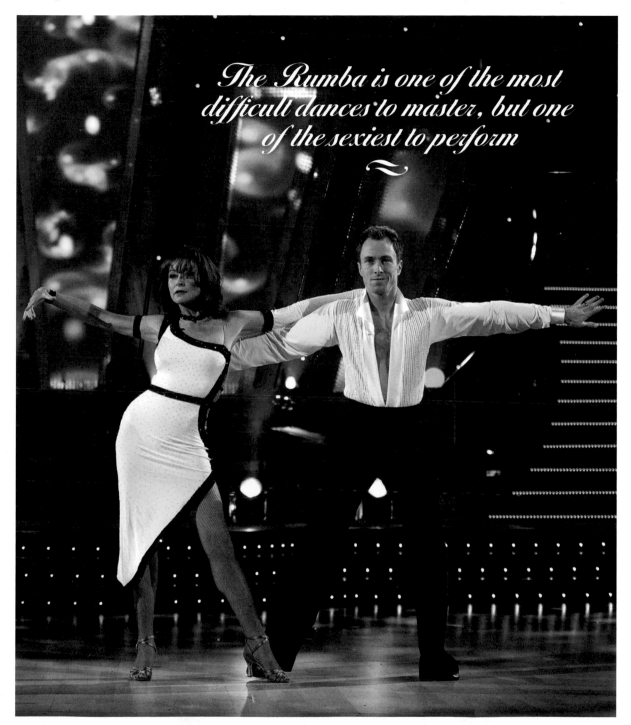

The Rumba is one of the most difficult dances to master, but one of the sexiest to perform

The Dance

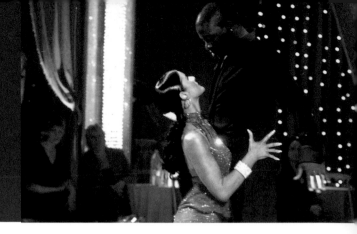

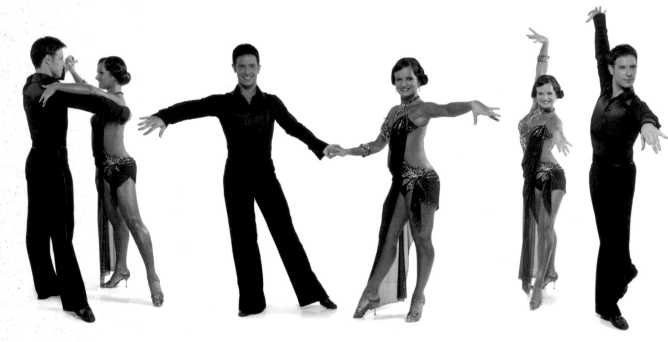

CLOSED HOLD
In this standard Latin hold, the points of contact are through his right arm with her left, and through the opposite hands. Bodies are toned, and there's a strong connection between the couple.

FAN POSITION
A basic Rumba step, showing the man and woman in an open position. The couple step apart, finishing at right angles to one another.

SLIDING DOORS
A figure with many variations. Here Darren and Lilia's lines are almost symmetrical – he's on his forward foot, she's on her back foot. The couple will then change places.

LEN'S OVERVIEW

What we're looking for in the Rumba is a connection between the couple. When Darren and Lilia dance the Rumba, they're looking at each other nearly all the time – and you can see the connection through their arms and hands. It's all about that contact. Look at the basic hold and you'll see that, although they're barely touching, they're still communicating. The Rumba should be romantic rather than sexy; it's all about the seduction and courtship. The man might be leading, but, if you look at the basic hold, you'll see that, in the Rumba, as in life, the girl always has the upper hand.

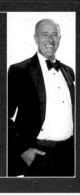

Rumba is a dance of romance, with the dancers expressing desire for each other. Technically, the couple has to be connected, disciplined and always showing elegant, extended lines.

TIMING

The Rumba rhythm is four beats, with one strong beat and three weak beats. In traditional music, a syncopated 'tock' sound can be heard, played on a pair of wooden sticks called 'claves'. For the dance timing, 'hold' (do not dance) for the first, strong beat, then step on beats 2, 3 and 4 of the music.

MUSIC

Romantic 4/4 music at 25 bars per minute is perfect for Rumba. Music can be either modern or Latin in mood. 'Chains' by Tina Arena, 'Mi Tierra' by Gloria Estefan and 'Jealous Guy' by Roxy Music are excellent Rumba dance tracks.

HOLD & POSTURE

The posture is upright, yet full of sinuous motion, especially in the hips. Arms are graceful and expressive, connected to the partner both in closed hold and single-hand hold.

LEGS & FEET

Strong foot pressure gives the dancers balance when moving slowly, and creates the sensuous Rumba hip action. Legs are toned to create long lines, and feet are pointed.

DRESS

A simple black silhouette for Darren, accentuating the line of the dance. Women's Rumba dresses are often revealing, expressing the sexual nature of the dance of seduction. Dramatic colours such as white, black and red are most appropriate.

OPENING OUT

The woman moves from the man's right side to his left in an open position. A classic Rumba move, this figure can be danced in a variety of rhythms.

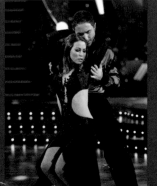

RUMBA DROP

One of the most spectacular moments in the dance, and a guaranteed crowd-pleaser. Despite the abandon of the pose, the line is extended from the tips of fingers to the end of toes.

The Steps

BASIC STEP
MAN'S STEPS

This figure is danced in closed hold.

Start with weight on right foot
1 Left foot forward (2)
2 Replace weight back on to right foot (3)
3 Left foot side (4) – hold (1)
4 Right foot back (2)
5 Replace weight forward on to left foot (3)
6 Right foot side (4) – hold (1)
End with weight on right foot
(Ball-Flat on all steps)

Note
This figure turns gently to left, and may turn up to ½ to left.

For all figures, 'hold' for beat 1 of music, then start dancing on beat 2.

BASIC STEP
LADY'S STEPS

Start with weight on left foot
1 Right foot back (2)
2 Replace weight forward on to left foot (3)
3 Right foot side (4) – hold (1)
4 Left foot forward (2)
5 Replace weight back on to right foot (3)
6 Left foot side (4) – hold (1)
End with weight on left foot
(Ball-Flat on all steps)

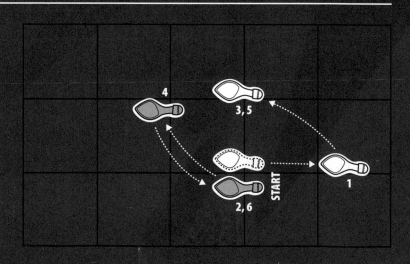

ALEMANA
MAN'S STEPS

This figure starts in closed hold.

Start with weight on right foot
1 Left foot forward (2)
2 Replace weight back on to right foot (3)
3 Left foot side, and lift left arm (4) – hold (1)
4 Right foot back (2)
5 Replace weight forward on to left foot (3)
6 Right foot side, and lower left arm when lady completes turn (4) – hold (1)
End with weight on right foot
(Ball-Flat on all steps)

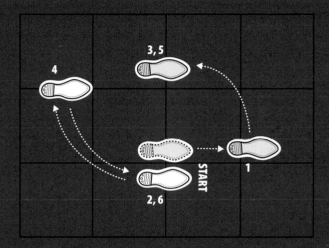

SUGGESTED AMALGAMATIONS

Basic Step – Alemana
Basic Step – Opening Out Right and Left
Basic Step – Alemana – Rope

ALEMANA
LADY'S STEPS

Start with weight on left foot
1 Right foot back (2)
2 Replace weight forward on to left foot (3)
3 Right foot side, and right arm is lifted (4) – hold (1)
4 Turn ⅛ to right, then left foot forward under raised arm (2)
5 Turn ½ to right, then right foot forward, stepping slightly away from man (3)
6 Turn ⅜ to right to face man, then left foot side (4) – hold (1)
End with weight on left foot
(Ball-Flat on all steps)

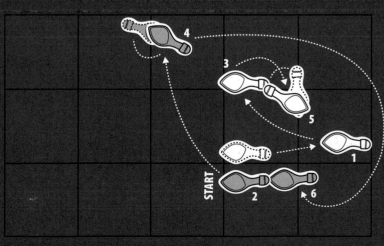

The Steps

OPENING OUT RIGHT AND LEFT
MAN'S STEPS

This figure starts and ends in closed hold.

Start with weight on right foot
1 Lead lady to turn ¼ to right, release left arm, then left foot side, keeping right foot in place (2)
2 Replace weight sideways on to right foot (3)
3 Lead lady to turn ¼ to left, taking closed hold with left arm, then left foot closes next to right foot (4) – hold (1)
4 Lead lady to turn ¼ to left, release right arm, then right foot side, keeping left foot in place (2)
5 Replace weight sideways on to left foot (3)
6 Lead lady to turn ¼ to right, resume closed hold, then right foot closes next to left foot (4) – hold (1)
End with weight on right foot
(Ball-Flat on all steps)

OPENING OUT RIGHT AND LEFT
LADY'S STEPS

Start with weight on left foot
1 Release right arm, then turn ¼ to right so that left side is near man, then right foot back (2)
2 Replace weight forward on to left foot (3)
3 Turn ¼ to left to face man, then right foot side and place right arm on man's left arm (4) – hold (1)
4 Release left arm, then turn ¼ to left so that right side is near man, then left foot back (2)
5 Replace weight forward on to right foot (3)
6 Turn ¼ to right to end facing man and resume closed hold, then left foot side (4) – hold (1)
End with weight on left foot
(Ball-Flat on all steps)

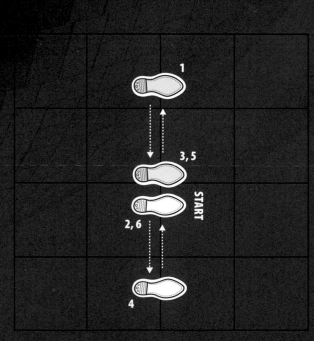

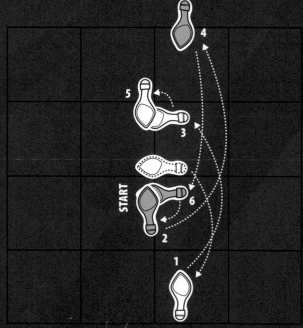

ROPE
MAN'S STEPS

This figure starts after step 6 of Alemana with lady facing man's right side.

Start with weight on right foot, left arm still raised from Alemana
1 Left foot side, keeping right foot in place (2)
2 Replace weight sideways on to right foot (3)
3 Left foot closes to right foot (4) — hold (1)
4 Right foot back (2)
5 Replace weight forward on to left foot (3)
6 Right foot side, and resume closed hold (4) — hold (1)
End with weight on right foot
(Ball-Flat on all steps)

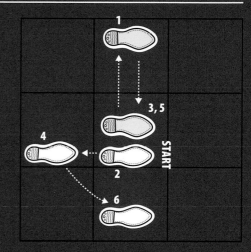

Note
Man circles left hand clockwise over his own head over steps 1–5, leading lady to walk clockwise around him.

ROPE
LADY'S STEPS

Start with weight to the side on left foot, right arm still raised from
    Alemana, facing man's right side
1 Right foot forward, start to walk in a clockwise circle around man (2)
2 Left foot forward (3)
3 Right foot forward, having made ½ turn clockwise around man (4)
    — hold (1)
4 Left foot forward (2)
5 Right foot forward (3)
6 Turn ¼ to right to face man, resume closed hold, then left foot side
    (4) — hold (1)
End with weight on left foot
(Ball-Flat on all steps)

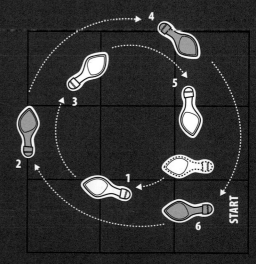

Note
Lady walks clockwise around man on steps 1–5.

Salsa

Hailing from the clubs of Cuba and Puerto Rico, Salsa is the least formal of all the dances. But, with its sexy hip movements, it's hotter than hell. Salsa has its roots in Samba, Rumba, Mambo and other African and Cuban dances. It's a playful yet risqué dance, expressed through the complex rhythms of Latin music. Salsa's compact movements reflect its origins in small dance clubs, where there wasn't much room for travelling steps. The name Salsa means 'sauce' and first appeared in the lyrics of a 1940s song about eating sausages! Now there are dozens of variations of this spicy dance from all over the Latin world.

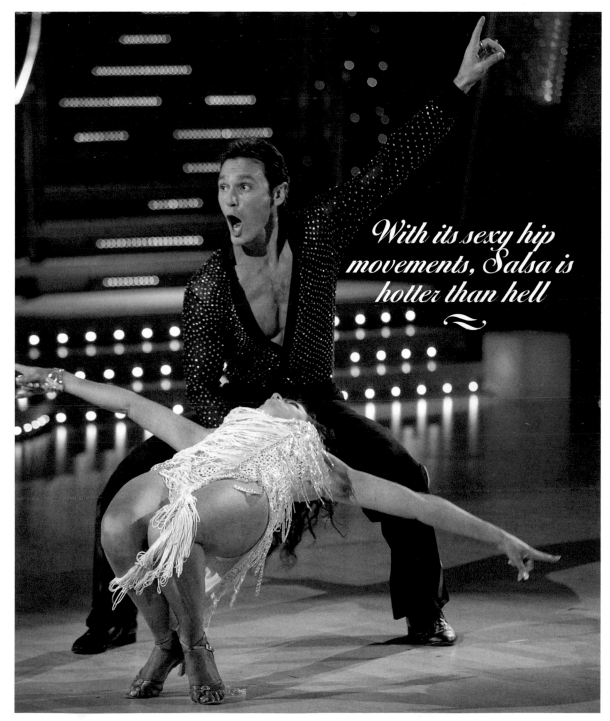

With its sexy hip movements, Salsa is hotter than hell

The Dance

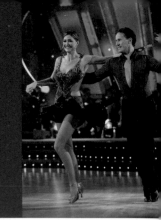

FORWARD AND BACK BASIC

The Forward and Back Basic form the foundation of 'New York' style Salsa. The man 'breaks' forward on the first beat and the woman 'breaks' back. Then the man 'breaks' back as the woman 'breaks' forward. This basic is very similar to the Rumba basic step, but with different timing.

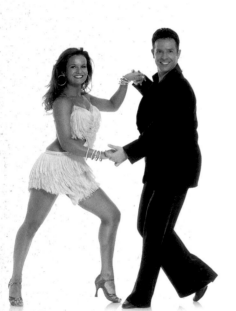

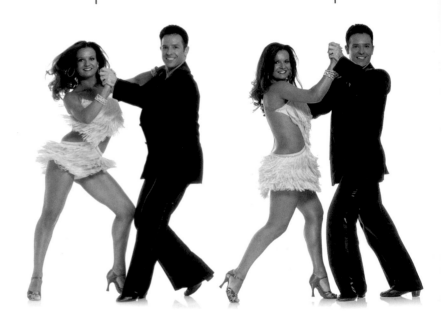

OPEN BASIC

Salsa is often danced in two-hand hold rather than the standard closed hold. This allows for easy transitions between complicated spins and drops.

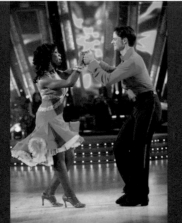

TURNING STEP

Darren and Lilia perform a turn with crossed hands, giving variety to underarm turns. In this hold, Darren can lead Lilia around behind him or spin her under his raised arms.

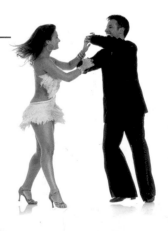

LEN'S OVERVIEW

One of the reasons I love Salsa is because it's the dance that the dance associations never got their hands on. It has kept its naturalness and spontaneity, rather than being formalized to death. I first came across it in Miami many years ago. At that time, Miami was full of illegal immigrants from Cuba, and they had the most fantastic clubs in a part of town that you'd never go to alone. Fortunately, I had a very good guide who took me to places that were full of young Cubans doing the sexiest dancing I had ever seen. It's basically a Rumba, but very fast — and, as it developed, it just got hotter and hotter. It remains a club dance, and the emphasis is on rhythm, rhythm, rhythm!

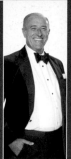

The emphasis is on sexy hip action, strong head movement, rapid footwork and quick-fire spins. As it's one of the faster Latin dances, Salsa will give you a good total body workout!

TIMING
Salsa music has four beats (one strong and three weak), but identifying the strong beat can take persistence, as Salsa music is renowned for its complexity. The dance has three steps danced over the four beats. For basic figures, dance on beats 1, 2 and 3, then 'hold' (don't dance) on beat 4.

MUSIC
'Ran Kan Kan' by Mambo great Tito Puente gets Salsa hips moving, as does Los Van Van's 'Cabeza Mala'. 'R&B Latino' by Alex Wilson gives Salsa a twenty-first-century sound.

HOLD & POSTURE
Salsa starts with the Latin closed hold, but quickly opens up into an enormous variety of holds and positions. Dancers may be quite casual in their posture, but they still require body tone — no slouching!

LEGS & FEET
The emphasis is on keeping the legs flexed and loose. The dancers stay close and low, giving a feeling of contained energy that bursts out through hip movement. The feet are the engine providing the rhythm, while the rest of the body makes all the sexy moves.

DRESS
The woman's dress shows as much flesh as possible. Fringing accentuates the hip movements. Men wear casual jackets and trousers, and open-necked shirts to keep the feel loose and informal.

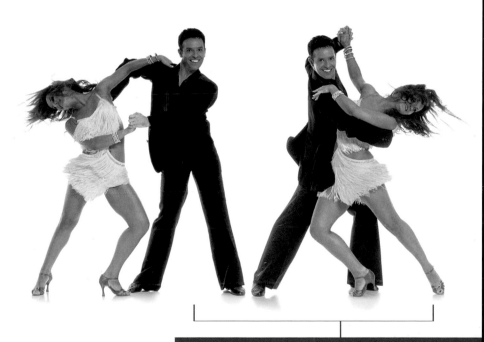

SCOOP
The woman hooks her left leg over his right, they maintain a strong hold and then he drops her in a sweeping semicircular motion from his right shoulder.

ROCKS
The man turns his partner out to right and left, keeping a strong hold and allowing her a full range of hip and head movements. In these flourishes, the Salsa really catches fire.

The Steps

BASIC STEP
MAN'S STEPS

This figure is danced in closed hold or two-hand hold.

Start with weight on right foot
1 Left foot forward (1)
2 Replace weight back on to right foot (2)
3 Left foot closes to right foot (3) – hold (4)
4 Right foot back (1)
5 Replace weight forward on to left foot (2)
6 Right foot closes to left foot (3) – hold (4)
End with weight on right foot
(Ball-Flat on all steps)

Note
This figure turns gently to left, and may turn up to ½ to left.

BASIC STEP
LADY'S STEPS

Start with weight on left foot
1 Right foot back (1)
2 Replace weight forward on to left foot (2)
3 Right foot closes to left foot (3) – hold (4)
4 Left foot forward (1)
5 Replace weight back on to right foot (2)
6 Left foot closes to right foot (3) – hold (4)
End with weight on left foot
(Ball-Flat on all steps)

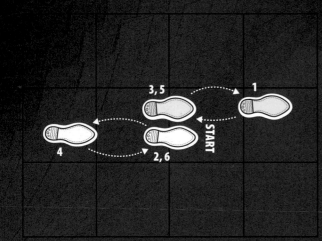

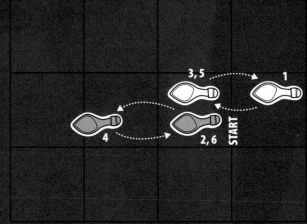

CROSS BODY LEAD
MAN'S STEPS

This figure is danced in closed hold.

Start with feet together, weight on left foot
1 Left foot forward (1)
2 Replace weight back on to right foot (2)
3 Turn ¼ to left, then left foot closes to right foot (3) – hold (4)
4 Right foot back (1)
5 Start turning to left, and replace weight forward on to left foot (2)
6 Right foot closes to left foot, having turned ¼ to left over steps 5–6 (3) – hold (4)
End with weight on right foot
(Ball-Flat on all steps)

CROSS BODY LEAD
LADY'S STEPS

Start with weight on left foot
1 Right foot back (1)
2 Replace weight forward on to left foot (2)
3 Right foot forward (3) – hold (4)
4 Left foot forward (1)
5 Turn ¼ to left, then right foot side (2)
6 Turn ¼ to left, then left foot back, ending facing man (3) – hold (4)
End with weight on left foot
(Ball-Flat on all steps)

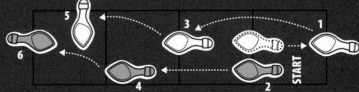

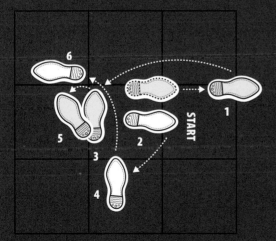

CROSS BODY LEAD – STEP 3

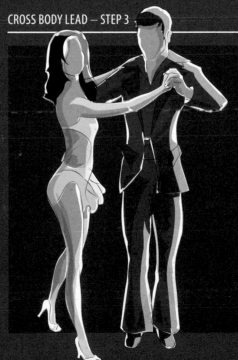

The Steps

OPEN BREAK AND UNDERARM TURN
MAN'S STEPS

This figure starts in closed or single-hand hold.

Start with weight on right foot
1 Release hold with right arm, then left foot back (1)
2 Replace weight forward on to right foot (2)
3 Left foot closes to right foot, and lift left arm (3) – hold (4)
4 Right foot back (1)
5 Replace weight forward on to left foot (2)
6 Right foot closes to left foot, and lower left arm when lady completes turn (3) – hold (4)
End with weight on right foot
(Ball-Flat on all steps)

Note
If next figure starts in closed hold, resume closed hold on steps 1–3 of next figure.

OPEN BREAK AND UNDERARM TURN
LADY'S STEPS

Start with weight on left foot
1 Release hold with left arm, then right foot back (1)
2 Replace weight forward on to left foot (2)
3 Right foot closes to left foot (3) – hold (4)
4 Turn ¼ to right, then left foot forward, keeping right foot in place (1)
5 Turn ½ to right, then replace weight forward on to right foot (2)
6 Turn ¼ to right to face man, then left foot closes to right foot (3) – hold (4)
End with weight on left foot
(Ball-Flat on all steps)

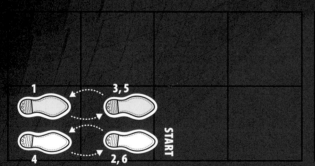

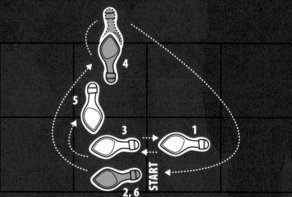

SUGGESTED AMALGAMATIONS

Basic Step – Cross Body Lead
Basic Step – Open Break and Underarm Turn
Basic Step – Open Break and Back Spot Turn
Basic Step – Cross Body Lead – Open Break and Underarm Turn
Basic Step – Cross Body Lead – Open Break and Back Spot Turn
Basic Step – Open Break and Back Spot Turn – Cross Body Lead

OPEN BREAK AND BACK SPOT TURN
MAN'S STEPS

This figure starts in closed hold or single-hand hold.

Start with weight on right foot
1 Release hold with right arm, then left foot back (1)
2 Replace weight forward on to right foot (2)
3 Resume closed hold, starting to turn to right, then left foot side (3) – hold (4)
4 Continuing to turn to right, right foot crosses behind left foot (1)
5 Continuing to turn to right, left foot side (2)
6 Right foot closes next to left foot, completing ¾ turn to right (3) – hold (4)
End with weight on right foot
(Ball-Flat on all steps)

OPEN BREAK AND BACK SPOT TURN
LADY'S STEPS

This figure starts in closed hold or single-hand hold.

Start with weight on left foot
1 Release hold with left arm, then right foot back (1)
2 Replace weight forward on to left foot (2)
3 Resume closed hold, starting to turn right, then right foot forward (3) – hold (4)
4 Continuing to turn to right, left foot forward (1)
5 Continuing to turn to right, right foot forward (2)
6 Left foot side, completing ¾ turn to right (3) – hold (4)
End with weight on left foot
(Ball-Flat on all steps)

Note
Figure may turn up to a total of one full turn over steps 3–6.

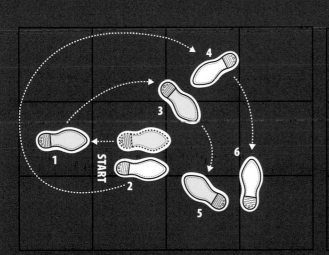

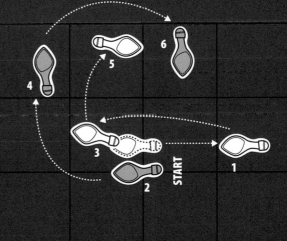

Viennese Waltz

The Viennese Waltz is a stately dance with relatively few steps, but requiring balance and stamina. It's all about rotation, with the couple continuously turning right and left in 3/4 time. While the Viennese Waltz is considered the height of sophistication, the dance actually has peasant origins. Its main antecedent is the Austrian Ländler, a dance in triple time that featured a great deal of hopping and stamping. The dance became faster and more refined as it moved into the ballrooms of the nineteenth century. Now, it's a chance for dancers to show that they're in tune as a couple, and have the strength to endure this whirling, elegant sprint.

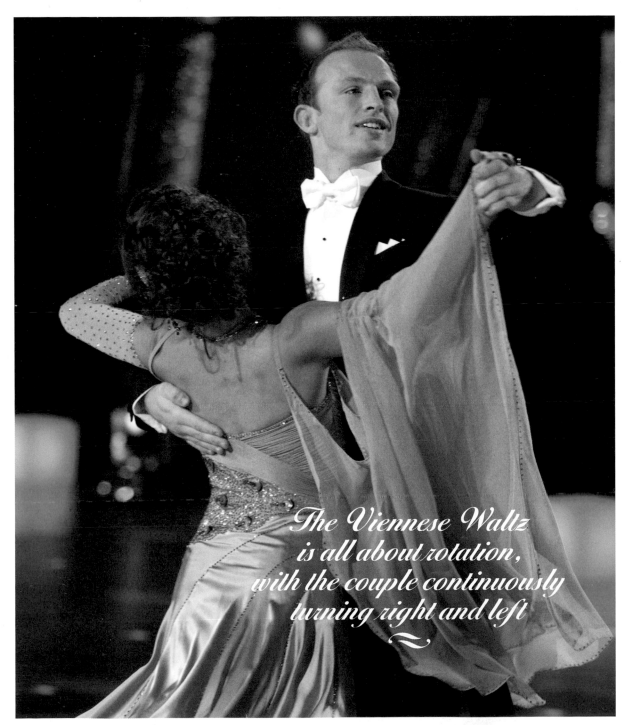

The Viennese Waltz
is all about rotation,
with the couple continuously
turning right and left

The Dance

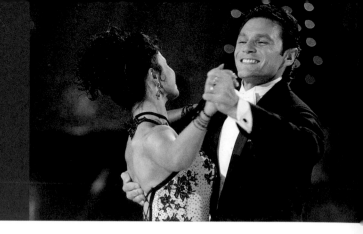

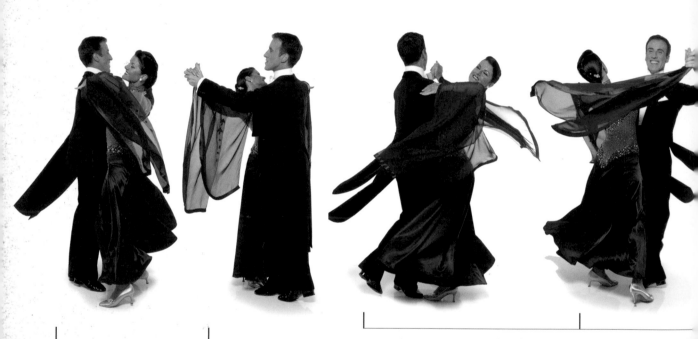

NATURAL TURN
The Natural Turn is a moving figure turning to the right, and on the third step both dancers close their feet.

REVERSE TURN
In the Reverse Turn the man crosses his left foot in front of his right on the third step, and the woman crosses on the sixth step.

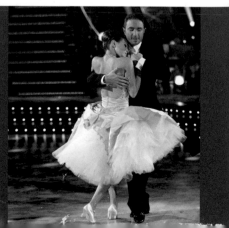

LEN'S OVERVIEW

The Viennese Waltz is most people's idea of ballroom dancing, and it's exhausting, like doing the 100-metre sprint, circling. There's nothing better than seeing dancers spinning around in one direction, then doing a quick Contra Check before they Fleckerl off the other way. This is the dance that you'd do to all those classic Strauss waltzes, like 'The Blue Danube'. It's the most limited of all the dances in terms of steps, so the hold and the technique have to be absolutely flawless.

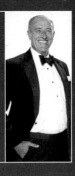

Viennese Waltz is the fastest of the ballroom dances. At 60 bars per minute, the dancers are taking 180 steps every minute – that's quite a workout!

TIMING

Viennese Waltz, like Waltz, has three beats – one strong beat and two weak beats. The rhythm has the classic 'Oom Pah Pah' sound. Steps 1 and 4 are danced on the strong beat, with the remaining steps danced on the weak beats.

MUSIC

While there are many classic Strauss Waltzes ('The Blue Danube' is the most recognizable), there are a lot of good modern Viennese Waltzes, including 'Que Sera Sera' (Doris Day), 'I Feel Pretty' (*West Side Story*) and the theme from the Harry Potter films.

HOLD & POSTURE

It's classic ballroom posture for this dance – the man is upright, while the woman arcs gracefully in his right arm. The hold must be toned and firm so that the dancers can successfully turn as one unit.

LEGS & FEET

Despite the apparent simplicity of the dance, the legs and feet are working hard. They must move very fast, dancing rise and fall without skipping, to give the dance its flowing quality.

DRESS

The skirt is full and flowing to emphasize the grace of the turn, while floating panels exaggerate the movement. Erin's midnight-blue dress with sparkling stones has a nocturnal feel.

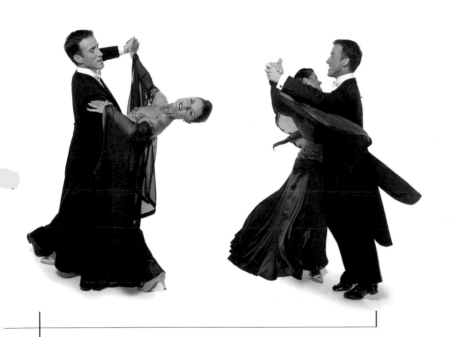

REVERSE FLECKERL, CONTRA CHECK & NATURAL FLECKERL

The Fleckerl is the most challenging figure in the Viennese Waltz. It is danced in the centre of the floor, and involves a complex pattern of side steps and crossing steps. After a number of Reverse (left-turning) Fleckerls, the dancers perform a Contra Check, giving them a graceful way to stop turning to the left. After the Contra Check, they begin rotating to the right. The challenge is to make a full turn every three steps, requiring the dancers to turn at dizzying speed.

The Steps

NATURAL TURN
MAN'S STEPS

This figure is danced in closed hold.

Start with weight on left foot
1 Turn ⅛ to right, then right foot forward (1)
2 Turn ¼ to right, then left foot side (2)
3 Turn ⅛ to right, then right foot closes to left foot (3)
4 Turn ⅛ to right, then left foot back (1)
5 Turn ⅜ to right, then right foot side (small step) (2)
6 Left foot closes to right foot (3)
End with weight on left foot (1. Heel-Toe, 2. Toe, 3. Toe-Heel, 4. Toe-Heel, 5. Toe, 6. Toe-Heel)

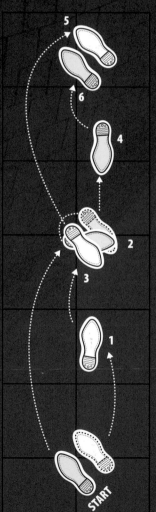

NATURAL TURN
LADY'S STEPS

Start with weight on right foot
1 Turn ⅛ to right, then left foot back (1)
2 Turn ⅜ to right, then right foot side (small step) (2)
3 Left foot closes to right foot (3)
4 Turn ⅛ to right, then right foot forward (1)
5 Turn ¼ to right, then left foot side (2)
6 Turn ⅛ to right, then right foot closes to left foot (3)
End with weight on right foot (1. Toe-Heel, 2. Toe, 3. Toe-Heel, 4. Heel-Toe, 5. Toe, 6. Toe-Heel)

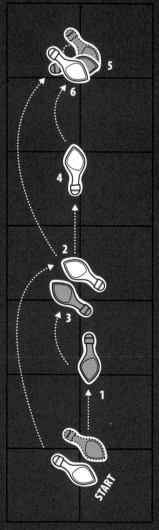

FORWARD CLOSED CHANGES
MAN'S STEPS

This figure is danced in closed hold.

Start with weight on left foot
1 Turn ⅛ to right, then right foot forward (1)
2 Turn ⅛ to right, then left foot side (2)
3 Right foot closes to left foot (3)
4 Turn ⅛ to left, then left foot forward (1)
5 Turn ⅛ to left, then right foot side (2)
6 Left foot closes to right foot (3)
End with weight on left foot
(1. Heel-Toe, 2. Toe,
3. Toe-Heel, 4. Heel-Toe,
5. Toe, 6. Toe-Heel)

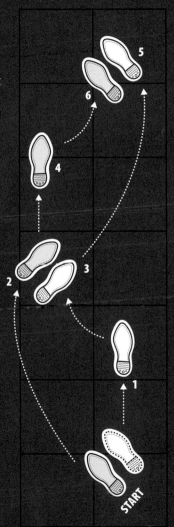

FORWARD CLOSED CHANGES
LADY'S STEPS

Start with weight on right foot
1 Turn ⅛ to right, then left foot back (1)
2 Turn ⅛ to right, then right foot side (2)
3 Left foot closes to right foot (3)
4 Turn ⅛ to left, then right foot back (1)
5 Turn ⅛ to left, then left foot side (2)
6 Right foot closes to left foot (3)
End with weight on right foot
(1. Toe-Heel, 2. Toe, 3. Toe-Heel, 4. Toe-Heel, 5. Toe, 6. Toe-Heel)

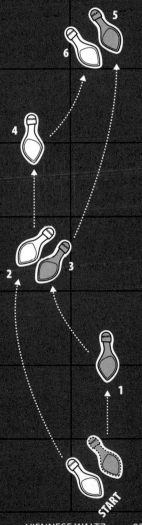

The Steps

REVERSE TURN
MAN'S STEPS

This figure is danced in closed hold.

Start with weight on right foot

1 Turn ⅛ to left, then left foot forward (1)

2 Turn ¼ to left, then right foot side (2)

3 Turn ⅛ to left, then left foot crosses in front of right foot (3)

4 Turn ⅛ to left, then right foot back (1)

5 Turn ⅜ to left, then left foot side (small step) (2)

6 Right foot closes to left foot (3)

End with weight on right foot
(1. Heel-Toe, 2. Toe, 3. Toe-Heel, 4. Toe-Heel, 5. Toe, 6. Toe-Heel)

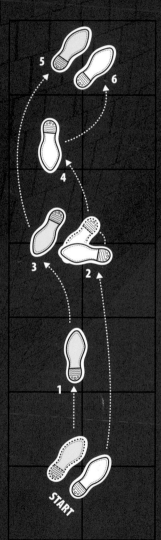

REVERSE TURN
LADY'S STEPS

Start with weight on left foot

1 Turn ⅛ to left, then right foot back (1)

2 Turn ⅜ to left, then left foot side (small step) (2)

3 Right foot closes to left foot (3)

4 Turn ⅛ to left, then left foot forward (1)

5 Turn ¼ to left, then right foot side (2)

6 Turn ⅛ to left, then left foot crosses in front of right foot (3)

End with weight on left foot
(1. Toe-Heel, 2. Toe, 3. Toe-Heel, 4. Heel-Toe, 5. Toe, 6. Toe-Heel)

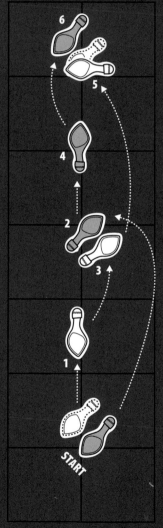

BACKWARD CLOSED CHANGES
MAN'S STEPS

This figure is danced in closed hold.

Start with weight on right foot

1 Turn ⅛ to right, then left foot back
2 Turn ⅛ to right, then right foot side (2)
3 Left foot closes to right foot (3)
4 Turn ⅛ to left, then right foot back (1)
5 Turn ⅛ to left, then left foot side (2)
6 Right foot closes to left foot (3)

End with weight on right foot
(1. Toe-Heel, 2. Toe, 3. Toe-Heel, 4. Toe-Heel, 5. Toe, 6. Toe-Heel)

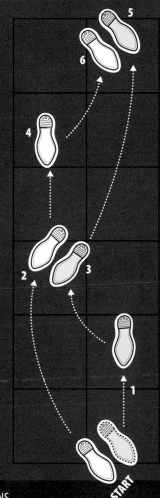

BACKWARD CLOSED CHANGES
LADY'S STEPS

Start with weight on left foot

1 Turn ⅛ to right, then right foot forward (1)
2 Turn ⅛ to right, then left foot side (2)
3 Right foot closes to left foot (3)
4 Turn ⅛ to left, then left foot forward (1)
5 Turn ⅛ to left, then right foot side (2)
6 Left foot closes to right foot (3)

End with weight on left foot
(1. Heel-Toe, 2. Toe, 3. Toe-Heel, 4. Heel-Toe, 5. Toe, 6. Toe-Heel)

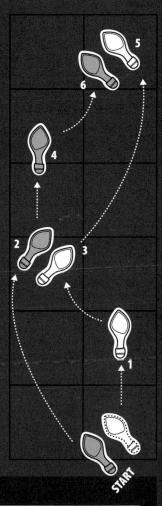

SUGGESTED AMALGAMATIONS

Natural Turn x 2 – Forward Closed Changes steps 1–3 – Reverse Turn x 2 – Forward Closed Changes steps 4–6

Natural Turn – Natural Turn steps 1–3 – Backward Closed Changes steps 1–3 – Reverse Turn steps 4–6 – Reverse Turn – Forward Closed Changes steps 4–6

Reverse Turn – Reverse Turn steps 1–3 – Backward Closed Changes steps 4–6 – Natural Turn steps 4–6 – Natural Turn – Forward Closed Changes steps 1–3

Samba

The Samba, a collision of African steps and Brazilian rhythms, is an exuberant feel-good dance. Hot Latin rhythms and wild movements give the real flavour of Mardi Gras and Carnival. The name of the dance derives from a Bantu word meaning 'to pray', and the dance and music originated as a way of calling forth the gods and inducing a trance in worshippers. The steps were modified in the nineteenth century and became popular in early twentieth century North America and Europe. This is a party dance, formalized for competitions but, even under strict rules, it retains its unrestrained nature.

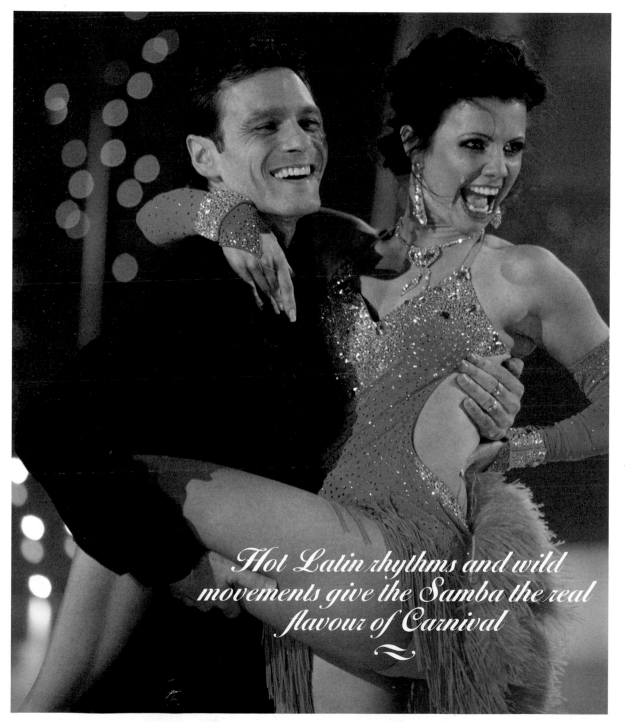

Hot Latin rhythms and wild movements give the Samba the real flavour of Carnival

The Dance

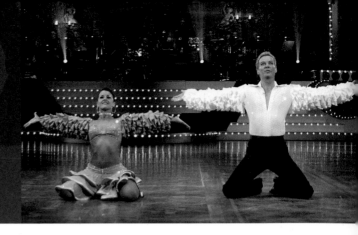

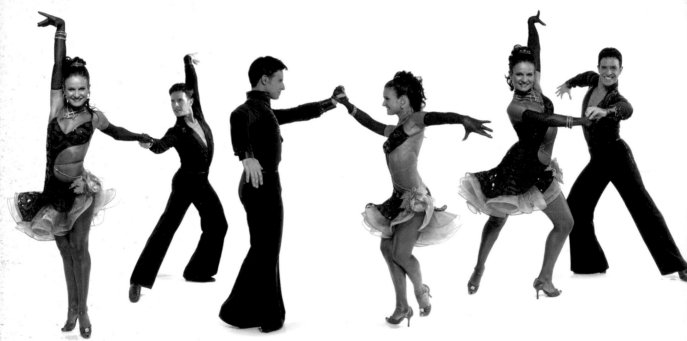

ROLLING OFF THE ARM
This figure's twirls and spins evoke the atmosphere of Brazilian Carnival. The woman rolls into the man's arms, then rolls out to side-to-side position, as the man dances Whisks.

VOLTA
This crossing action of the feet can be danced either in a straight line (as demonstrated), in a circle or on the spot.

CRISS-CROSS BOTAFOGOS
The Botafogo was named after Botafogo Bay in Brazil. The dancer moves side to side, settling on to a soft knee with the opposite leg extended. Here Lilia crosses in front of Darren.

LEN'S OVERVIEW

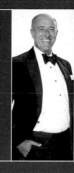

When you watch the Samba you should be transported to Rio de Janeiro for Carnival. Samba music makes everybody want to move their hips, and that's really what it's all about. The fluidity of the hips gives rhythm to the legs, whether you're travelling or dancing on the spot. A good Samba performance is very sexy. It's not like the seduction of the Rumba; it's much more flirtatious and teasing.

Samba should have the flavour of a wild party, with sexy costumes, bright colours and up-tempo music. But be warned: the judges are still looking for technique beneath the sizzling surface!

TIMING
The rhythm of Samba music is '1-a-2, 1-a-2'. Beat 1 is strong, beat 2 is weak. Both beats could be classified as 'slows'. When dancing Samba, the 'a' step comes ¾ of the way between the first and second beats. The Volta is danced over four beats, with 'a' steps in between the beats.

MUSIC
Samba's basic '1-a-2' rhythm has many variations, but the 50–52 bars per minute music should make you want to bounce. Super tracks include 'Brazil' (Xavier Cugat), 'Half a Minute' (Matt Bianco) and 'Hips Don't Lie' (Shakira).

HOLD & POSTURE
Samba requires suppleness and strength, and a flexible spine for Samba Rolls. Arms must remain toned for a good connection with a partner when dancing at high speed.

LEGS & FEET
Samba is danced with a distinct bounce in the standing knee. The foot placement, knee bounce and hips accentuate the rhythm of the music.

DRESS
Another case of 'less is more'. Women wear cut-away party outfits in bright colours with short skirts, allowing the focus to be on the limbs. If the man's in good shape, out comes the chest!

SHADOW ROLL
The couple are in full body contact as their upper bodies 'roll' either clockwise or anticlockwise. Here, Darren and Lilia show Reverse Samba Rolls in shadow position.

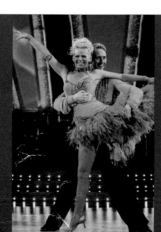

PROMENADE RUNS
Another fast-moving figure, in which the dancers take turns crossing in front of each other as they travel across the floor. Spins and pivots are sometimes added to give extra excitement.

The Steps

WHISKS
MAN'S STEPS

This figure is danced in closed hold.

Start with weight on right foot
1 Left foot side (1)
2 Right foot crosses behind left foot (a)
3 Replace weight forward on to left foot (2)
4 Right foot side (1)
5 Left foot crosses behind right foot (a)
6 Replace weight forward on to right foot (2)
End with weight on right foot
(1. Ball-Flat, 2. Ball, 3. Ball-Flat, 4. Ball-Flat, 5. Ball, 6. Ball-Flat)

Notes
It is recommended to repeat steps 1–6 before going on to another figure.

To follow Whisks with Samba Walks, man turns ⅛ to left and lady turns ⅛ to right on steps 5–6 to end in promenade position.

WHISKS
LADY'S STEPS

Start with weight on left foot
1 Right foot side (1)
2 Left foot crosses behind right foot (a)
3 Replace weight forward on to right foot (2)
4 Left foot side (1)
5 Right foot crosses behind left foot (a)
6 Replace weight forward on to left foot (2)
End with weight on left foot
(1. Ball-Flat, 2. Ball, 3. Ball-Flat, 4. Ball-Flat, 5. Ball, 6. Ball-Flat)

For all steps with the timing 'a', step on the ball of the foot only, keeping the heel raised.

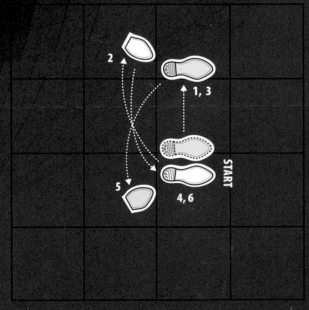

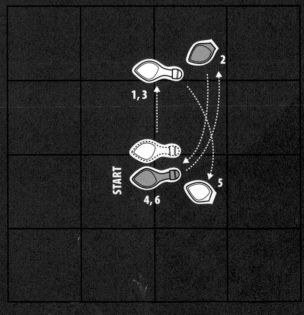

SAMBA WALKS
MAN'S STEPS

This figure is danced in promenade position.

Start with weight forward on right foot
1 Left foot forward (1)
2 Replace weight back on to right foot (a)
3 Replace weight forward on to left foot (2)
4 Right foot forward (1)
5 Replace weight back on to left foot (a)
6 Replace weight forward on to right foot (2)
End with weight on right foot
(1. Ball-Flat, 2. Ball, 3. Ball-Flat, 4. Ball-Flat, 5. Ball, 6. Ball-Flat)

Note
It is recommended to repeat steps 1–6 before going on to another figure.

SAMBA WALKS
LADY'S STEPS

Start with weight forward on left foot
1 Right foot forward (1)
2 Replace weight back on to left foot (a)
3 Replace weight forward on to right foot (2)
4 Left foot forward (1)
5 Replace weight back on to right foot (a)
6 Replace weight forward on to left foot (2)
End with weight on left foot
(1. Ball-Flat, 2. Ball, 3. Ball-Flat, 4. Ball-Flat, 5. Ball, 6. Ball-Flat)

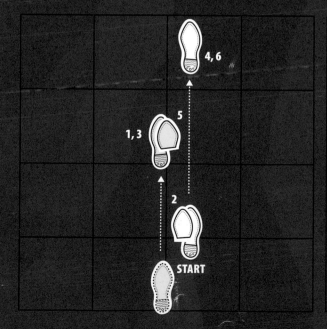

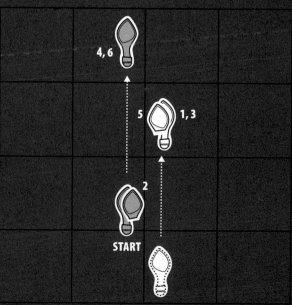

The Steps

VOLTAS
MAN'S STEPS

This figure is danced in closed hold.

Start with weight on left foot
1 Right foot forward and across (1)
2 Left foot side (small step) (a)
3 Right foot crosses in front of left foot (2)
4 Left foot side (small step) (a)
5 Right foot crosses in front of left foot (3)
6 Left foot side (small step) (a)
7 Right foot crosses in front of left foot (4)
End with weight on right foot
(1. Ball-Flat, 2. Ball, 3. Ball-Flat, 4. Ball, 5. Ball-Flat, 6. Ball, 7. Ball-Flat)

VOLTAS
LADY'S STEPS

Start with weight on right foot
1 Left foot forward and across (1)
2 Right foot side (small step) (a)
3 Left foot crosses in front of right foot (2)
4 Right foot side (small step) (a)
5 Left foot crosses in front of right foot (3)
6 Right foot side (small step) (a)
7 Left foot crosses in front of right foot (4)
End with weight on left foot
(1. Ball-Flat, 2. Ball, 3. Ball-Flat, 4. Ball, 5. Ball-Flat, 6. Ball, 7. Ball-Flat)

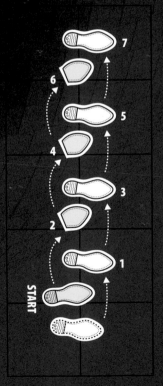

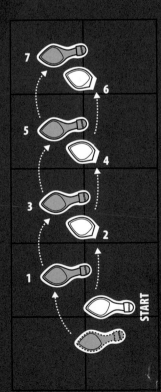

SUGGESTED AMALGAMATIONS

Whisks x 2 – Samba Walks x 2 – Whisks

Whisks x 2 – Samba Walks – Samba Walks steps 1–3 – Voltas – Whisks

Whisks x 2 – Samba Walks – Samba Walks steps 1–3 – Botafogos in Promenade and Counter-Promenade Positions x 2 – Samba Walks steps 4–6 – Whisks

BOTAFOGOS IN PROMENADE AND COUNTER PROMENADE
MAN'S STEPS

This figure starts and ends in promenade position.

Start with weight on left foot
1 Right foot forward (1)
2 Turn ⅛ to right to face lady, loosening right arm hold, then left foot side (a)
3 Turn ⅛ to right into counter promenade position, then replace weight on to right foot (2)
4 Left foot forward and across in counter-promenade position (1)
5 Turn ⅛ to left to face lady, returning right arm to closed hold, then right foot side (a)
6 Turn ⅛ to left to promenade position, then replace weight on to left foot (2)

End with weight on left foot
(1. Ball-Flat, 2. Ball, 3. Ball-Flat, 4. Ball-Flat, 5. Ball, 6. Ball-Flat)

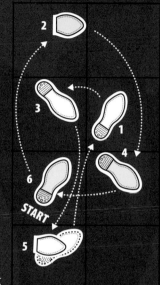

Note
It is recommended to repeat steps 1–6 before dancing another figure. If repeating steps 1–6, maintain loosened hold until figure is completed.

BOTAFOGOS IN PROMENADE AND COUNTER PROMENADE
LADY'S STEPS

Start with weight on right foot
1 Left foot forward (1)
2 Turn ⅛ to left to face man, loosening left arm hold, then right foot side (a)
3 Turn ⅛ to left into counter promenade position, then replace weight on to left foot (2)
4 Right foot forward and across in counter-promenade position (1)
5 Turn ⅛ to right to face man, returning left arm to closed hold, then left foot side (a)
6 Turn ⅛ to right to promenade position, then replace weight on to right foot (2)

End with weight on right foot
(1. Ball-Flat, 2. Ball, 3. Ball-Flat, 4. Ball-Flat, 5. Ball, 6. Ball-Flat)

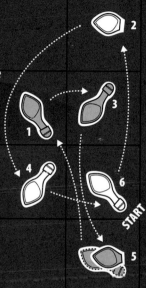

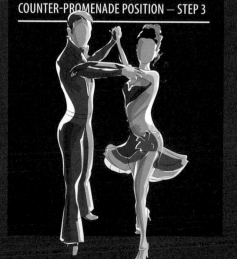

COUNTER-PROMENADE POSITION — STEP 3

Waltz

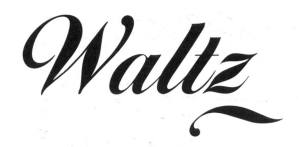

The Waltz is considered the epitome of elegance, but there was a time when this dance was regarded as scandalous. When the Viennese Waltz, one of the precursors of the Waltz, reached England in the late eighteenth century, it was immediately denounced in polite society because of the sustained body contact between the dancers. The Waltz retains this element of body contact, and the *Strictly* judges are keen to see the couple move 'as one'. The nearest ancestor to today's 'slow' Waltz is the Hesitation Waltz, made famous in the 1920s in America by the great dancers Vernon and Irene Castle.

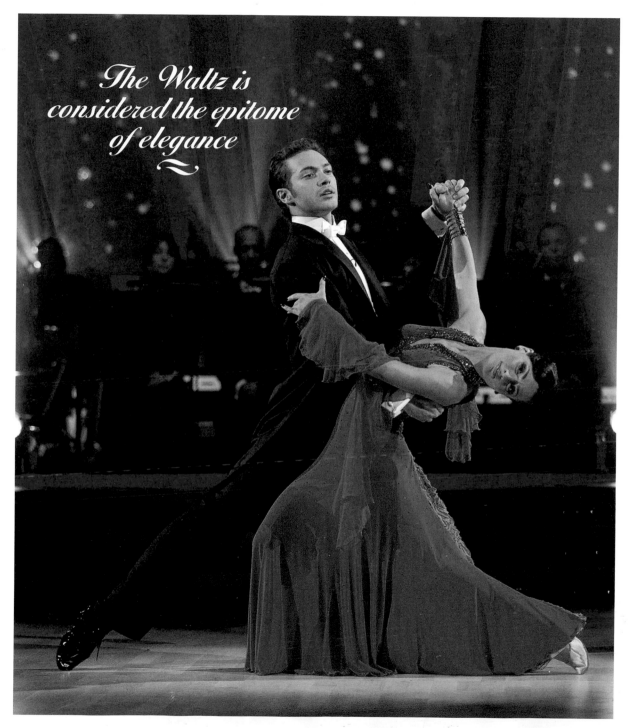

The Waltz is considered the epitome of elegance

The Dance

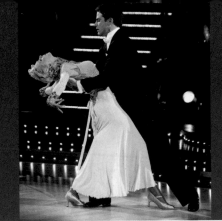

THROWAWAY OVERSWAY
The man dances around in front of the woman before turning her, guiding her left leg back, and allowing her body to extend backward in an elegant curve.

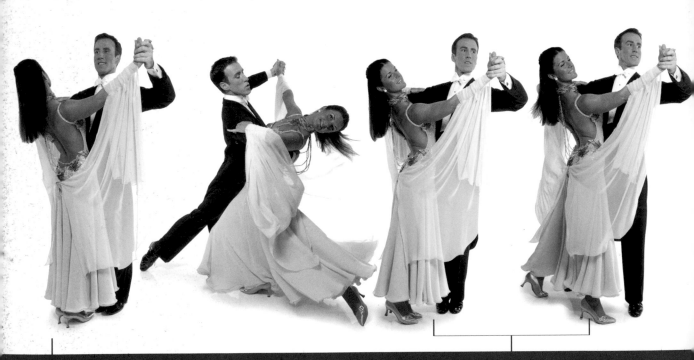

BALLROOM HOLD
The woman is slightly to the man's right side. His right hand is on her back near the shoulder blade, and her left hand is placed on his right upper arm (above and inset).

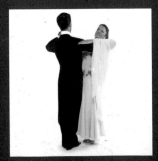

PROMENADE
A basic ballroom action in which both dancers are moving forward. The bodies are still in contact but in a slight V-shaped position.

LEN'S OVERVIEW

A Waltz should flow. It has a rise and fall, a lyrical, musical feeling that should be magical to watch. To an audience, it appears to float on a cloud – but it's all in that basic ballroom hold. The man's posture must be erect and vertical and, whatever shapes the couple get into, they must maintain all the points of contact. But they're touching, not clinging – there should always be a lightness about it. You have to be very strong and supple to do all those turns and Overswrays, but the discipline is hidden by the magic and romance of the movement. It's an illusion.

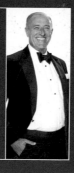

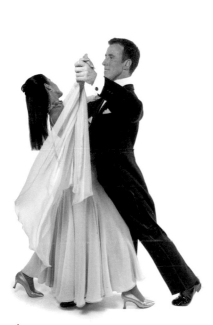

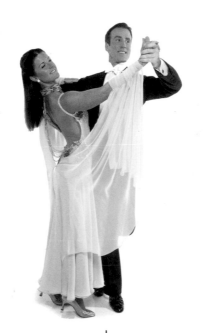

Performing a good rise and fall requires strong leg and foot muscles, while core strength helps maintain the full body contact and synchronize movements with one's partner.

TIMING
Like Viennese Waltz music, the slow Waltz has three beats. The first beat is strong, the second and third beats weak. Steps 1 and 4 are danced on the strong beat, with the remaining steps danced on the weak beats. The Chassé (steps 4—7 of the Whisk & Chassé) has the timing '12&3' - the '&' beat comes half way between beats 2 and 3.

MUSIC
'Moon River' is one of the best-known classic Waltzes, while 'Come Away With Me' by Norah Jones captures the romantic feel. The music is played in 3/4 time at 29—30 bars per minute.

HOLD & POSTURE
No matter what variations the dancers perform, the basic hold remains constant throughout the dance. Each dancer must support his or her own arms so as not to weigh down their partner.

LEGS & FEET
There is rise and fall throughout the Waltz, with the dancers bending their knees and going up on the toes, giving the dance a soft, wave-like quality.

DRESS
Classic white tie and tails for the man — the uniform for nearly all ballroom dances. The woman wears a light, floating dress, accentuating the softness of her movement.

NATURAL TURN
'Natural' indicates a right turn ('reverse' is a left turn), commencing with the man's right foot forward. Body contact remains constant, with no space between the hips.

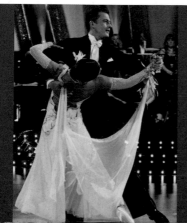

WHISK
On the third step the dancers' feet end in a crossed position, and the bodies and heads are in promenade position.

The Steps

CLOSED CHANGES
MAN'S STEPS

This figure is danced in closed hold.

Start with weight on left foot
1 Right foot forward (1)
2 Left foot side (2)
3 Right foot closes to left foot (3)
4 Left foot forward (1)
5 Right foot side (2)
6 Left foot closes to right foot (3)
End with weight on left foot
(1. Heel-Toe, 2. Toe, 3. Toe-Heel, 4. Heel-Toe, 5. Toe, 6. Toe-Heel)

Note
When dancing Closed Changes only, dance with man moving forward around the floor. When danced in conjunction with other figures, the direction of the Closed Changes will be dictated by the direction of the other figures.

CLOSED CHANGES
LADY'S STEPS

Start with weight on right foot
1 Left foot back (1)
2 Right foot side (2)
3 Left foot closes to right foot (3)
4 Right foot back (1)
5 Left foot side (2)
6 Right foot closes to left foot (3)
End with weight on right foot
(1. Toe-Heel, 2. Toe, 3. Toe-Heel, 4. Toe-Heel, 5. Toe, 6. Toe-Heel)

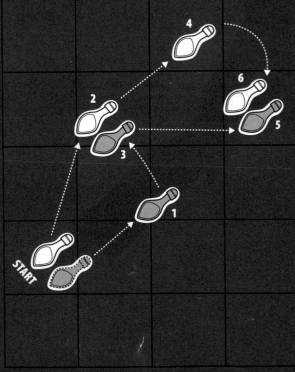

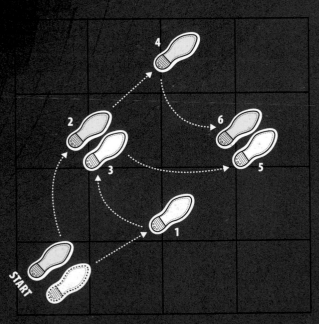

NATURAL TURN
MAN'S STEPS

This figure is danced in closed hold.

Start with weight on left foot
1 Right foot forward (1)
2 Turn ¼ to right, then left foot side (2)
3 Turn ⅛ to right, then right foot closes to left foot (3)
4 Left foot back (1)
5 Turn ⅜ to right, then right foot side (2)
6 Left foot closes to right foot (3)
End with weight on left foot
(1. Heel-Toe, 2. Toe, 3. Toe-Heel, 4. Toe-Heel, 5. Toe, 6. Toe-Heel)

NATURAL TURN
LADY'S STEPS

Start with weight on right foot
1 Left foot back (1)
2 Turn ⅜ to right, then right foot side (2)
3 Left foot closes to right foot (3)
4 Right foot forward (1)
5 Turn ¼ to right, then left foot side (2)
6 Turn ⅛ to right, then right foot closes to left foot (3)
End with weight on right foot
(1. Toe-Heel, 2. Toe, 3. Toe-Heel, 4. Heel-Toe, 5. Toe, 6. Toe-Heel)

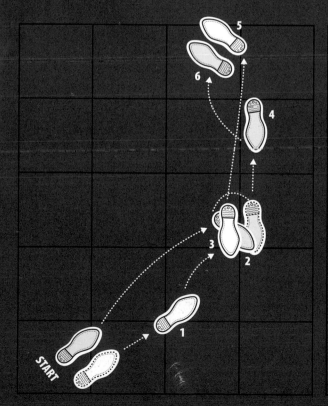

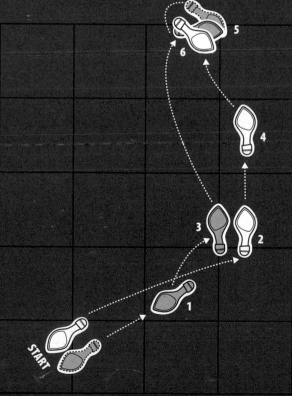

The Steps

REVERSE TURN
MAN'S STEPS

This figure is danced in closed hold.

Start with weight on right foot
1 Left foot forward (1)
2 Turn ¼ to left, then right foot side (2)
3 Turn ⅛ to left, then left foot closes to right foot (3)
4 Right foot back (1)
5 Turn ⅜ to left, then left foot side (2)
6 Right foot closes to left foot (3)
End with weight on right foot
(1. Heel-Toe, 2. Toe, 3. Toe-Heel,
4. Toe-Heel, 5. Toe, 6. Toe-Heel)

REVERSE TURN
LADY'S STEPS

Start with weight on left foot
1 Right foot back (1)
2 Turn ⅜ to left, then left foot side (2)
3 Right foot closes to left foot (3)
4 Left foot forward (1)
5 Turn ¼ to left, then right foot side (2)
6 Turn ⅛ to left, then left foot closes to right foot (3)
End with weight on left foot
(1. Toe-Heel, 2. Toe, 3. Toe-Heel,
4. Heel-Toe, 5. Toe, 6. Toe-Heel)

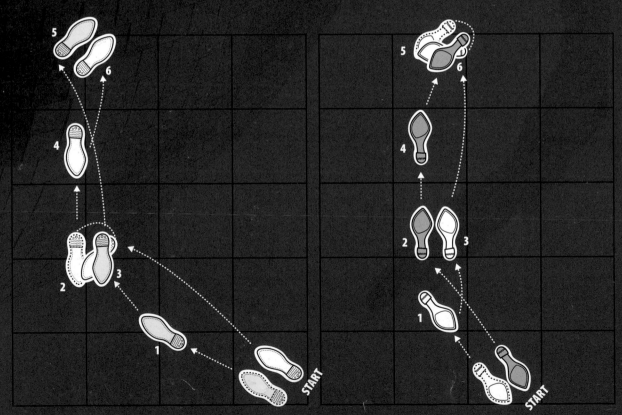

WHISK AND CHASSÉ
MAN'S STEPS

This figure is danced in closed hold.

Start with weight on right foot
1 Left foot forward (1)
2 Right foot side, turning shoulders to right (2)
3 Left foot crosses behind right foot in promenade position (3)
4 Right foot forward and across in promenade position (1)
5 Left foot side, turning shoulders to left to resume original hold (2)
6 Right foot closes to left foot (&)
7 Left foot side (3)
End with weight on left foot
(1. Heel-Toe, 2. Toe, 3. Toe-Heel, 4. Heel-Toe, 5. Toe, 6. Toe, 7. Toe-Heel)

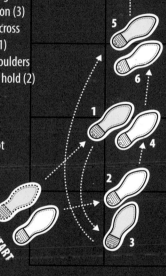

WHISK AND CHASSÉ
LADY'S STEPS

Start with weight on left foot
1 Right foot back (1)
2 Left foot side (2)
3 Turn ¼ to right, then right foot crosses behind left foot in promenade position (3)
4 Left foot forward and across in promenade position (1)
5 Turn ⅛ to left, resume original hold, then right foot side (2)
6 Turn ⅛ to left, then left foot closes to right foot (&)
7 Right foot side (3)
End with weight on right foot
(1. Toe-Heel, 2. Toe, 3. Toe-Heel, 4. Heel-Toe, 5. Toe, 6. Toe, 7.Toe-Heel)

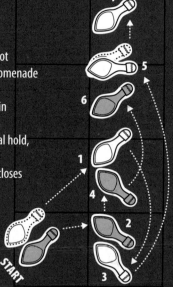

Note
The first step of the next figure will be danced outside partner.

SUGGESTED AMALGAMATIONS

Closed Changes progressing anticlockwise around dance floor
Natural Turn – Closed Changes steps 1–3 – Reverse Turn
    – Closed Changes steps 4–6
Natural Turn – Closed Changes steps 1–3 – Reverse Turn
    – Whisk and Chassé

WHISK AND CHASSÉ – STEP 3

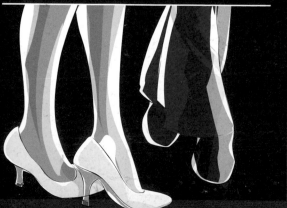

OUT NOW

The Official 2010 Annual

To buy books by your favourite authors and
register for offers, visit

www.rbooks.co.uk

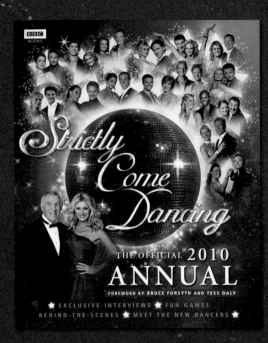

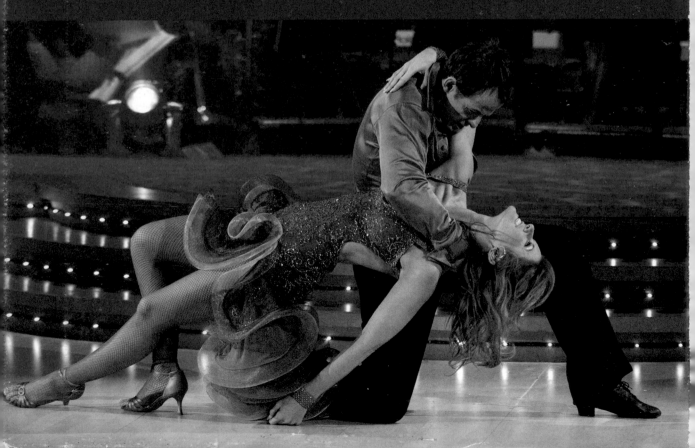